CAN DEATH BE A HARM TO THE PERSON WHO DIES?

Philosophy and Medicine

VOLUME 73

The titles published in this series are listed at the end of this volume

CAN DEATH BE A HARM TO THE PERSON WHO DIES?

by

JACK LI

Fooyin Institute of Technology, Taiwan

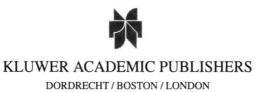

KLUWER ACADEMIC PUBLISHERS

DORDRECHT / BOSTON / LONDON

A C.I.P. Catalogue record for this book is available from the Library of Congress.

ISBN 1-4020-0505-9

Published by Kluwer Academic Publishers,
P.O. Box 17, 3300 AA Dordrecht, The Netherlands.

Sold and distributed in North, Central and South America
by Kluwer Academic Publishers,
101 Philip Drive, Norwell, MA 02061, U.S.A.

In all other countries, sold and distributed
by Kluwer Academic Publishers, Distribution Center,
P.O. Box 322, 3300 AH Dordrecht, The Netherlands.

Printed on acid-free paper

Printed in the Netherlands.

For my wife
Tsui-Chu

CONTENTS

Preface	ix
Introduction	1
1. The Epicurean Argument	11
1.1 Explication of the Epicurean Argument	11
1.2 A Critique of the Epicurean Argument	19
2. The Desire-thwarting Theory	33
2.1 Explication of the Desire-thwarting Theory	33
2.2 Shortcomings of the Desire-thwarting Theory	37
3. The Deprivation Theory	43
3.1 Explication of the Deprivation Theory	43
3.2 A Critique of the Deprivation Theory	48
4. The Interest-Impairment Theory	67
4.1 Interests and Harms	67
4.2 The Harms of the Death Event and Premature Death	74
4.3 Posthumous Harms and the Missing Subject Problem	82
4.4 The Timing of the Harm of Death	88
5. The Lucretian Symmetry Argument	99
5.1 Explication of the Lucretian Symmetry Argument	99
5.2 The Failure of the Lucretian Symmetry Argument	101
5.3 Fear of Death	124
Conclusion	131
Notes	139
Bibliography	179
Index	191

PREFACE

It is with great pleasure that I write this preface for Dr Li's book, which addresses the venerable and vexing issues surrounding the problem of whether death can be a harm to the person who dies. This problem is an ancient one which was raised long ago by the early Greek philosopher Epicurus, who notoriously argued that death is at no time a harm to its 'victim' because before death there is no harm and after death there is no victim.

Epicurus's conclusion is conspicuously at odds with our prereflective—and in most cases our post-reflective—intuitions, and numerous strategies have therefore been proposed to refute or avoid the Epicurean conclusion that death cannot be an evil after all. How then are we to account for our intuition that death is not just an evil, but perhaps the worst evil that may befall us? This is the key issue that Dr Li addresses.

Dr Li's book explores various alternative approaches to the complex and difficult issues surrounding Epicurus's notorious argument and provides a defence of the intuitively plausible conclusion that death can indeed be a harm to the person who dies. This challenge to Epicurus's claim that death is never a harm to the person who dies is developed by way of a detailed exploration of the issues raised not only by Epicurus, but also by his many successors, who have responded variously to the challenging issues which Epicurus raised. Dr Li's book is a valuable contribution to, and continuation of, a debate which has stimulated philosophical reflection for millennia.

On a personal note I have known Dr Li for many years and have worked closely with him on these problems, which he first addressed as a postgraduate research student in philosophy at the University of Queensland where he successfully completed his PhD under my supervision. I have high regard for the quality of Dr Li's philosophical abilities and achievements and it is therefore with great pleasure that I welcome the publication of this book to disseminate his arguments more widely to the global community of philosophical scholars.

William Grey, PhD (Cambridge)
Associate Professor of Philosophy
University of Queensland

INTRODUCTION

It is popularly believed that death is the most terrifying of ills. Besides, death is a matter of ultimate concern for each of us—everyone will directly face it *sooner or later*. But no one, while still alive, can ever experience it. This might be part of the reason why death has appeared as a riddle or mystery (or even an inexpressible beauty) to many human beings. Given this, it should not be any surprise that death has long been addressed in a variety of inquiries: religion (or theology), psychology, medicine, and literature. Of course, *philosophy* is among these. Death in fact is a vitally important topic in philosophy. Plato (427-437 B.C.) even insisted that, '...those who really apply themselves in the right way to philosophy are directly and of their own accord preparing themselves for dying and death.'[1]

There are many *philosophical* puzzles pertaining to death. Some of them relate to moral problems such as euthanasia or abortion. Others are related to metaphysical problems, which are relatively more basic and abstract. There are important connections between metaphysical and moral questions. In this book, however, I will not focus on these moral issues. Rather, I will investigate one of the more basic and abstract problems concerning the nature of death: *'Can death be a harm to the person who dies?'* (To this question, my answer is, 'Yes!')

In exploring the reason for the affirmative answer to this question, I want to avoid getting involved in not only a variety of religious, psychological or even medical issues about death, but also various moral issues about death. In particular, I do not want to deal with the issue over whether there is a soul[2], or whether there is an afterlife.[3] I will just assume that there is no soul (and no afterlife). In contrast, I will assume that death is complete annihilation. That is, when dead, the very person has permanently ceased to exist.

Although most people regard death as a great harm to be avoided, Epicurus (341-270 B.C.) tells us that death is *nothing to us*. The most powerful part of his argument for this conclusion can be put as follows:

In order to be harmed, a person must be in existence at the time. But death is the cessation of one's existence which is beyond harm or gain. Thus, death cannot be a harm.[4]

This argument can be expressed as follows:

> (1) No harm can befall one who does not exist.
> (2) Death is complete annihilation. When dead, one does not exist.
> (3) Thus, no harm can befall one who is dead.
> (4) Therefore, death cannot be a harm.

Although Epicurus' argument is untenable (as we will see in Chapter One, Section Two), he *does* however raise a very serious challenge for the position on the other side—the 'missing subject problem'. In a very important sense, any theory attempting to justify the badness of death (e.g. the deprivation theory) is merely a reply to (or the resolution of) the missing subject problem. To justify the claim that death can be a harm to the person who dies, of course, it is necessary for me to resolve the missing subject problem. In this book, in justifying the badness of death, I will focus on the resolution of the missing subject problem.

For the purpose of the discussions later, it is important to have an appropriate understanding of the concept of death. It is useful therefore to distinguish the notion 'dying' from the notion 'death'. Put simply, dying is the process whereby one comes to be dead. When a person is dying, he[5] is still alive. Apparently, dying can involve significant pain and suffering. Thus, it is not particularly puzzling why dying can be a harm to a person, insofar as pain and suffering can certainly be a harm to an individual. On the other hand, death is an experiential blank.[6] But what exactly is 'death'?

According to John Martin Fischer, there are three different approaches to illustrating or exposing the concept(s) of (human) death: (1) the biological approach, (2) the moral approach, and (3) the metaphysical approach. With respect to the biological approach, Fischer writes:

> [The biological] approach takes the relevant or significant aspects of human life to be those in virtue of which we are *organisms* of a certain kind. The proponents of this approach attempt to derive illumination about death from the notion that it is particularly significant that humans are organisms of a certain sort.[7]

He describes the moral approach as follows:

> [The moral approach] is to seek illumination of human death by reference to moral intuitions about when it is justifiable to regard and treat a person as dead.[8]

As to the metaphysical approach, Fischer says:

> [The metaphysical] approach to elucidating human death proceeds via metaphysical considerations. Specifically, one version of this approach claims that an adequate understanding of the nature and criteria of personal identity will lead to an appropriate account of human death.[9]

For one to have a deeper and more comprehensive understanding of the notion of death, it is necessary to investigate all the issues related to these three approaches. However, since I want to focus on the missing subject problem, I will not discuss all these issues. For the purpose of the discussion in this book, I think it is enough to define 'death' as *the permanent and irreversible cessation of one's existence.*

This definition can be interpreted in terms of consciousness (or psychology) or biology. Some philosophers, however, insist that death should be defined as the termination of conscious (or mental) life but not the termination of biological life.[10] For convenience, I will ignore the issue of whether death should be defined that way or not. I will simply suppose that whenever the termination of conscious (or mental) life happens, the termination of biological life happens as well.

It is important to identify at the outset six assumptions which will be made throughout this book:

1. I presuppose that life (or being alive) is *generally* good.

2. The word 'bad' has come to be used by some authors, such as Fischer, as a synonym for 'harm'; this usage of an adjective as a noun may grate on the ears of some readers. However, the prevalence of this usage has made it difficult to avoid in the discussion that follows. In fact, the following four concepts—'harm', 'misfortune', 'evil', or 'bad'—are slightly different. It seems that 'evil' is full of the flavour of religion or mystery. On the other hand, 'misfortune' seems to be subjective, comparing with 'harm'. And the badness of death, as we will see, is an objective matter. Thus, I think 'harm' is the best term to choose among these four. However, for convenience, I will not distinguish between them, except to note a difference between 'bad' and the rest of them in terms of degree. For example, 'harm' ('misfortune', or 'evil') suggests a more serious 'bad', whereas 'bad' suggests a slight 'harm' ('misfortune', or 'evil').

3. In this book, I want to justify the badness of *death*, but not the badness of dying. That is to say, what I am concerned about is the state of being dead, but not the process of dying.

Some philosophers, like Stephen E. Rosenbaum, believe that, apart from these two stages, there is a third stage intervening between dying and death (being dead). This stage takes place at the end of dying and the beginning of death (being dead).[11] To deal with the various problems (or issues) related to this stage would divert me from the main path. Indeed, it is certainly not an easy task to deal with all these issues. For example, it is not clear whether or not this stage exists. Nor is it clear whether or not it takes time (if it *does* exist). In order to focus on the resolution of the missing subject problem, I will just presuppose that there is *no* such stage.

Even if this stage exists, I, in making this presupposition, still do not miss the point. For even in this situation, I can, by showing that death (being dead) can be a harm to a person, still prove that this stage can be a harm as well. That is, I can prove that all three stages can be harms. The reason for this is as follows. Evidently, dying can be a harm. If I can establish that death, which is farther from dying in time, can also be a harm, then it would be false to claim that this stage, which is closer to dying in time, cannot also be a harm.

4. By 'the death event', I mean a process following from the cause of death to death (being dead). No doubt, it is very likely that one would feel discomfort or even experience some pain in this process. One could be tortured to death, or otherwise made to suffer before his death (being dead). However, it should be emphasised here that, while defining a death event as above, I do not include the possible harm or evil one might suffer in this process. So described, a death event could be considered as equivalent to a *painless* process leading to death (being dead).

It is clear that death (being dead) is the state of affairs directly brought about by the death event. Given that the death event is understood in this way, the following conclusion can be reached: If the death event is not a harm to a person, then death (being dead) should not be a harm to him either; whereas if the death event is a harm to him, then death (being dead) must be a harm to him as well. In contrast, if death (being dead) is not a harm to him, then the death event should not be a harm to him either; whereas if death (being dead) is a harm to him, then the death event must be a harm to him as well.

In fact, it makes no difference whether we say death (being dead) is a harm (or not a harm) or the death event is a harm (or not a harm).[12] However, the characteristics of the death event are clearer and thus, more easily grasped. That is to say, it is easier for us to discuss or investigate the relevant issues or questions by using the notion of the death event. Given this, instead of using 'death' (being dead), I will mostly use 'the death event' in the following discussion.

5. Some philosophers, such as Jeff McMahan, have suggested that personal identity is a matter of degree. If so, then death is also a matter of degree.[13] While I take this point, in order to concentrate on the missing subject problem, I will presuppose that personal identity is not a matter of degree, and thus the temporal boundaries of birth and death will be assumed to be quite sharp.

6. According to the Epicurean argument, death is not a harm even to a young person. To simplify discussion, by 'death' in this book I mean the premature cessation of life unless otherwise indicated.

It should be emphasised here that the purpose of this book is to justify the claim that death can be a harm to the person who dies. If there is an afterlife, then clearly death can be a harm. For we can imagine a peculiarly terrifying state in our afterlife in which we somehow continue to exist and hence suffer. In other words, if we presuppose that there is a soul, then we can justify this claim easily. On the other hand, if we presuppose that there is no soul, then this claim would meet a very difficult challenge from Epicurus as shown above—the missing subject problem. My book is an argument against the missing subject problem, so I assume that there is no soul. In sum, I make these assumptions purely for the sake of argument, not because I necessarily think that they are true.

Now, let me outline the structure of this book.

The Epicurean argument concludes that death is *never* a harm to the person who dies. Most philosophers have attempted (often unsuccessfully) to reject this conclusion. The Epicurean conclusion directly contradicts the conclusion I will reach in this book—death *can* be a harm to the person who dies. My first objective will therefore be to reject the Epicurean argument. If successful, then I can claim that it is possible for death to be a harm to the person who dies. This would, undoubtedly, be a big step towards my objective.

The Epicurean argument is indeed incorrect: the essential and most powerful premise in this argument is the Existence Requirement—a person *can* be the subject of some harm or misfortune *only if* he exists at the time the harm or misfortune occurs. However, this premise is incorrect. Therefore, the Epicurean argument should be rejected, as I will argue in Chapter One.

The claim that death can be a harm to the person who dies requires some justification. There are two main theories which try to justify this claim: the 'desire-thwarting theory' and the 'deprivation theory'. The desire-thwarting theory can be briefly expressed as follows:

> (1) Something is a harm or misfortune for us if it thwarts any of our desires.
> (2) Death thwarts certain kind(s) of our *unconditional* desires.
> (3) Therefore, death is a harm or misfortune for us.[14]

On the other hand, the deprivation theory can be simply put as follows:

> Death is a harm for the person who dies because it deprives him of certain goods—the goods he would have enjoyed if he had not died.[15]

I will discuss these two theories in Chapters Two and Three respectively. In Chapter Two, I shall endeavour to show that the desire-thwarting theory is problematic. I will argue that the desire-thwarting theory is an unacceptable theory, because, roughly, the concept of desire is too *subjective*, so the thwarting of desire fails to present the characteristics of harm (or badness)—including, of course, the harm (or badness) of death. On the other hand, although the concept of 'the deprivation (or loss) of goods' is objective enough, I shall undertake to show, in Chapter Three, that the deprivation theory still has its limitations. Let me explain.

As we will see in Chapter Three, Section Two, when considering the case of a person, P, who dies prematurely, we can, and usually *do*, take two very different perspectives:

> (1) P's death event (or the event which brings about P's death) is a harm to him.

(2) P's premature death (or the fact that P dies prematurely)[16] is a
harm to him.

Although these two notions are very different, they are closely related. For
one thing, in the present case P's death event will certainly bring about his
premature death. On the other hand, if we claim that P can be harmed by his
own death event, then it is natural for us also to claim that he can be harmed
by a variety of posthumous events. I will support the widely held view that
these two claims are so related that we are obliged either to affirm both or to
deny both.[17]

Accordingly, in the case of a person who dies prematurely, the following
three notions are strongly connected: 'the badness of his premature death (or
the badness of the fact that he dies prematurely)', 'the badness of his death
event (or the badness of the event which brings about his death)', and 'his
posthumous harms'. However, the deprivation theory can, as I will show,
explain only the badness of his death event. This suggests that there might be
scope for a new comprehensive theory which can explain: (1) why a person's
premature death (or the fact that a person dies prematurely) is *always* a harm
to him; (2) why a person's death event (or the event which brings about a
person's death) can be a harm to him; and (3) why a person can be harmed
posthumously. The deprivation theory might be a component of the
comprehensive theory. This is the task of Chapter Four.

To meet this task, I want first, in Chapter Four, Section One, to illustrate
the concept of harm in order to really grasp the meanings of these three
questions above. In other words, I want to show that 'harm' is best defined as
the impairment of (objective) interest (I call this the 'interest-impairment
principle'). On the basis of this principle, I shall endeavour further to explore,
in Chapter Four, Sections Two and Three, a theory (which I call the
'interest-impairment theory') to justify the following claims: (1) a person's
death event (or the event which brings about a person's death) can be a harm
to him, (2) a person's premature death (or the fact that a person dies
prematurely) is *always* a harm to him, and (3) a person can be harmed
posthumously.

So far, I have outlined the nature of the harm of death (if it is a harm at all).
To have a more complete answer to the question, 'Can death be a harm to the
person who dies?', it is still necessary to sort out two relevant puzzles which
are raised in particular by Epicureans.

The first is this. If death can harm a person, *who* is the subject of the harm?
In other words, if the person is no longer alive, how can *he* be the subject of

the harm?

The second is as follows. *When* does the harm occur? Can a harm take place after its subject ceases to exist? It seems that it cannot. After all, it appears there cannot be harm without a subject to be harmed. If so, then it seems that the harm must take place before its subject ceases to exist. However, this seems to be difficult to accept as well. After all, before death, the harm event has not yet occurred.

The first puzzle is the missing subject problem. This 'problem' will be dealt with in Chapter Four, Section Three. Then, I shall undertake to sort out the second puzzle of the timing of the harm of death in Chapter Four, Section Four. I will argue that the subject of the harm of death is the *ante-mortem* person—*the once living person who is no longer with us*. And, the timing of the (subject's) harm of death must be *before death*.

If I can identify the nature of the harm of death and if I can also resolve these two puzzles, then I can confidently conclude that *death can be a harm to the person who dies.*

In Chapter Five I go on to consider some arguments developed by Lucretius (c. 99-55 B.C.). Following Epicurus, Lucretius addresses himself to proving that death is *never* a harm so it is never rational now for us to be bothered by death.[18] His argument—the Lucretian symmetry argument—can be very simply put as this:

(1) No one is bothered by prenatal nonexistence.
(2) Posthumous nonexistence is metaphysically analogous to prenatal nonexistence (the symmetry thesis).
(3) Therefore, we should not be bothered by the prospect of posthumous nonexistence.

The Lucretian symmetry argument is usually juxtaposed with the discussion of the Epicurean argument (discussed in Chapter One). However, the discussion of the Lucretian symmetry argument necessarily involves the consideration of the nature of the badness of death (especially the deprivation theory). For a more perspicuous discussion, I have therefore located it in Chapter Five.

Apparently, the Lucretian symmetry argument endeavours to prove the following two conclusions:

(i) Neither prenatal nonexistence nor death is a harm.

(ii) It is not rational for us to fear either our death or our prenatal nonexistence now.

No doubt, Lucretius' conclusion (i) would directly challenge the conclusion I want to reach in this book—*death can be a harm to the person who dies*. Hence, to secure my position, it is necessary for me to reject the Lucretian symmetry argument.

It is clear that (i) has theoretical priority over (ii). For only if we determine whether death is a harm and whether prenatal nonexistence is a harm, can we properly consider the appropriate attitudes toward these two periods. Thus, to reject the Lucretian symmetry argument, it is better and easier to focus on (i). That is, the *symmetry thesis* is the crucial premise in the Lucretian symmetry argument. Logically speaking, there are three possible approaches to rejecting the symmetry thesis:

(1) Showing that prenatal nonexistence is a harm, but death is not a harm.
(2) Showing that both prenatal nonexistence and death are harms.
(3) Showing that prenatal nonexistence is not a harm, but death is a harm.

These three positions can be called: (i) Prenatal harm approach, (ii) Prenatal-and-Posthumous harm approach, (iii) Posthumous harm approach.

In Chapter Five, I will discuss these three positions. I want to show that the first two positions are incorrect. Although the Posthumous harm approach is correct, I shall argue that there are some versions of this approach which are problematic and thus, cannot be accepted either—the 'metaphysical personal identity version' (suggested by Thomas Nagel[19]) and the 'psychological version' (suggested by Frederik Kaufman[20]). I will go on to outline the best way to reject the symmetry thesis.

Given that the symmetry thesis is incorrect, the Lucretian symmetry argument should be rejected. If so, then the conclusion we will have reached in Chapter Four—*death can be a harm to the person who dies*—will be undisturbed.

Given this conclusion, it seems reasonable to claim that the fear of death is rational. However, this claim might be challenged as follows:

Even if death is a harm, it is still irrational to fear death. For the fear of death cannot change the fact that we will die eventually.[21]

This issue will be explicated and discussed in Chapter Five, Section Three. I will argue: If 'death' is understood as premature death, then it is rational to fear it; whereas if 'death' is understood as necessary mortality, then it is irrational to fear it.

Finally, in Conclusion, I will provide a brief review and indicate some direction for further study.

CHAPTER ONE

The Epicurean Argument

The Epicurean argument has provided the classical objection to the widely held view that death can be a harm to the person who dies. To attain the central aim of this book, first of all, I want to refute Epicurus in this chapter.

I do not want to die—no; I neither want to die nor do I want to want to die; I want to live for ever and ever and ever.

--Miguel de Unamuno, *Tragic Sence of Life*

The common-sense view of death, as Harry S. Silverstein explains, is that a person's death is one of the greatest evils that can befall him.[1] However, Epicurus[2], in his paper "Letter to Menoeceus", develops a famous argument about death to challenge this common-sense view. Epicurus writes:

> Become accustomed to the belief that death is nothing to us. For all good and evil consists in sensation, but death is deprivation of sensation…So death, the most terrifying of ills, is nothing to us,

since so long as we exist death is not with us; but when death comes, then we do not exist. It does not then concern either the living or the dead, since for the former it is not, and the latter are no more.[3]

Call this the 'Epicurean argument'.

Put simply, the main point of the Epicurean argument is:

Death cannot be a harm or misfortune for the person who dies, for, when death occurs, there is no longer a subject to whom any harm or misfortune can be ascribed.[4]

It is quite apparent that according to the Epicurean argument, the answer to the question, 'Can death be a harm to the person who dies?' is simply, 'No!'

The Epicurean argument can be reconstructed as follows:

(A) A state of affairs (or event) is a harm (or bad thing) for someone P *only if* P can experience it.

(B) Therefore, P's death is a harm to P *only if* it is a state of affairs that P can experience.

(C) P can experience a state of affairs *only if* it begins before P's death.

(D) P's death is not a state of affairs that begins before P's death.

(E) Therefore, P's death is not a state of affairs that P can experience.

THEREFORE, P's death is not a harm to P.[5]

This reconstruction (which I call the 'standard interpretation of the Epicurean argument'[6]), with an appropriate (and I believe correct) understanding of the Epicurean argument, not only offers a clearer philosophical expression to the Epicurean argument, but also makes explicit some notions implicit in the Epicurean argument.[7] Therefore, I believe that we thereby get a clearer and deeper understanding of the Epicurean argument.

For the rest of this section, I want to explicate the Epicurean argument and its standard interpretation.

1. The Epicurean argument does not rule out that our deaths are harms to others or someone else's death is a harm to us. It could be argued, for example, that my death can be a source of misery to others, especially to my family.

2. For an appropriate understanding of the Epicurean argument, it is very important to distinguish two concepts from each other:

> (1) Dying—the process whereby one comes to be dead or the process wherein certain causes operate to bring about one's death.
> (2) Death—the permanent and irreversible cessation of one's existence. Intuitively it is the state which one is in at and after one dies. In a word, death is 'being dead'. In this state there is apparently no subject left.

Dying takes place during a person's lifetime and, apart from the terminal stage, may thus be experienced. That is, when one is dying, one is still alive. On the other hand, death (being dead) is clearly not part of a person's life. If someone P died at T then his dying preceded T, whereas his death occurred at T and after T the subject is dead.[8]

There is no doubt that the conclusion of the Epicurean argument concerns *death (being dead)*, and not dying. The reasons for this are:

(i). It is very clear that a person's dying can be a harm to him, as Fischer states:

> When one is dying, one is still alive. One can be conscious of dying, and dying can involve significant pain and suffering. It is not particularly puzzling why dying can be a bad thing for a person, insofar as pain and suffering can certainly be bad for an individual.[9]

(ii). In his argument, Epicurus says, '...when we are, death is not, and when death is come, we are not...' Here, what Epicurus talks about is a state of affairs which is temporally located when *we are not*. However, dying takes place during our lifetime. That is, when dying comes, we still are.

Therefore, the conclusion of the Epicurean argument does not rule out a person's dying being a harm to him.[10]

Some philosophers believe that there is a stage intervening between dying and death (being dead). This stage takes place at the end of dying and the beginning of death (being dead).[11] If this stage *does* exist, then another issue arises: *'Is the conclusion of the Epicurean argument also about the stage intervening between dying and death (being dead)?'* or *'Does the conclusion of the Epicurean argument rule out the stage intervening between dying and death (being dead)?'*

Rosenbaum, who believes that there is a stage intervening between dying and death (being dead), gives two reasons to refute the idea that the conclusion of the Epicurean argument is about the stage between dying and death (being dead):

(1) Construing Epicurus as taking 'death' to be a sort of tertiary period in one's history would be an exceedingly uncharitable way of making him look silly.
(2) The issue would be much less interesting if it concerned this tertiary period instead of death (being dead). What people seem to think as bad is not the moment of this tertiary period itself, but rather the abysmal nonexistence of being dead. This, at any rate, is what they fear, and that fear is what Epicurus wished to extinguish.[12]

Someone, who also believes that there is a stage intervening between dying and death (being dead), might try to reject Rosenbaum's argument as follows:

Although it is very clear that the conclusion of the Epicurean argument is not concerned with dying, it is not clear that it is concerned only with being dead. Epicurus might use only the term 'death' to refer to both 'the stage intervening between dying and being dead' and 'being dead'. In other words, the conclusion of the Epicurean argument might be concerned not only with being dead, but also with the stage intervening between dying and being dead. There is no reason to expect Epicurus to have thoughtfully distinguished between these two concepts and to have selected the Greek equivalent of 'being dead' to express his view. From these two reasons, what Rosenbaum can justify is only that, 'The conclusion of the Epicurean argument cannot be concerned *only* with this tertiary period' or "It is incorrect to take the term 'death' in the Epicurean argument to be *only* a sort of tertiary period in one's history." Indeed, from his two reasons, Rosenbaum cannot show that the stage intervening between dying and being dead cannot be a part of 'death' in Epicurus' sense.

This criticism sounds reasonable. If it is accepted, then Rosenbaum fails to show that the conclusion of the Epicurean argument rules out the stage intervening between dying and being dead. We now face a difficulty in judging or deciding whether 'death' in the Epicurean argument covers a stage intervening between dying and being dead. We should not expect to sort out this difficulty by considering *only* the Epicurean argument itself. We need also to consider some related factors.

The characteristics of the stage intervening between dying and being dead (if this stage exists) are still unclear. According to Rosenbaum, this stage is roughly the time at which a person becomes dead. However, it is not clear that it is a part of a person's lifetime. It is not clear that it takes time or, if so, how much time it takes. It may be a mere moment in time separating dying from being dead.[13] Most importantly, it is not clear whether or not there is a subject left during this stage; nor is it clear, if there is a subject during this stage, what the characteristics of this subject are or in what sense it is a subject at all. Perhaps for this reason, Julian Lamont uses a strange circumlocution to call the subject (if we can call it 'subject') during this stage: 'qua presently living subject'.[14] These unclear factors about the characteristics of this stage are partly responsible for our hesitation in judging or deciding whether 'death' in the Epicurean argument covers a stage intervening between dying and being dead (if this stage exists).

For the following reasons, I will suppose that 'death' in the Epicurean argument does not cover a stage intervening between dying and being dead.

(i). The essential characteristic of 'death' in the Epicurean argument is 'of no subject'. It is because of this characteristic that Epicurus concludes that 'death' (in Epicurus' sense) cannot be a harm to the person who dies. Thus, to Epicurus, 'no subject' is a criterion for 'death' in a very important sense. This stage is different from dying and being dead in some way. Otherwise, it would be nonsense to claim: 'There is a stage intervening between *dying* and *being dead*'. It is clear that, if one is in a state of 'being dead', then there is no subject left. Since this stage is different from 'being dead', it might not be appropriate to claim that, if one is in this stage, then there is no subject left. It might be more appropriate to say that there is a 'semi subject' left during this stage. If this is the case, then, according to Epicurus' criterion for death, it is not appropriate to count this stage (with a semi *subject*) as death.

(ii). If this stage is of 'no subject' (which is very improbable), then, according to Epicurus' criterion for death, 'death' in the Epicurean argument would cover both being dead and this stage. In this case, being dead is part of 'death' in the Epicurean argument, so there is no problem for Epicurus to agree the claim that death (being dead) cannot be a harm to the person who dies. Of course, he might add that, 'Well, this stage cannot be a harm to the person who dies either'. However, for the purpose of this book, even if 'death' in the Epicurean argument would cover both being dead and this stage, it is enough to suppose that 'death' in the Epicurean argument covers only being dead. The reasons for this are as follows.

The purpose of this book is to justify the claim that death (being dead) can be a harm to the person who dies. In his argument, Epicurus concludes that 'death' (in his sense) cannot be a harm to the person who dies. If we suppose that 'death' in the Epicurean argument does not cover this stage, then his conclusion would be: Death (being dead) cannot be a harm to the person who dies. In this case, if I can reject Epicurus, then I can at least affirm the possibility that death (being dead) can be a harm to the person who dies.

In fact, once I can prove the possibility that death (being dead) can be a harm to the person who dies, I can also prove the possibility that this stage can be a harm. The reason for this is as follows.

Clearly dying can be a harm. If it is possible for death (being dead) (which is farther from dying in time) to be a harm, then it would be false to claim that it is impossible for this stage (which is closer to dying in time) to be a harm.

Of course, to attain the purpose of this book, it is still all right to suppose that 'death' in the Epicurean argument covers this stage. However, the cost for doing this would be very high. To completely reject the Epicurean argument, we need to deal with the problematic issues about the characteristics of this stage. This could take a lifetime as there appears no chance of reaching definitive answers to these issues. Let alone it is possible that there is in fact no stage intervening between dying and being death.

Accordingly, I will therefore assume that the conclusion of the Epicurean argument rules out the stage intervening between dying and death (being dead).

3. The conclusion of the Epicurean argument does not rule out that the anticipation of our own deaths can be a harm to us. Firstly, while this anticipation happens, we are still alive. It is quite obvious that such anticipation can be a harm to us, for it can disturb us. Secondly, Epicurus uses the fact of death's not being a harm to us to argue that the prospect of our own death *should not* disturb us. He writes:

...the man speaks but idly who says that he fears death not because it will be painful when it comes, but because it is painful in anticipation. For that which gives no trouble when it comes, is but an empty pain in anticipation.[15]

It is clear that for most people the prospect of their own death, Epicurus observes, is disturbing, and he attempts to lessen this unease. In short, the conclusion of the Epicurean argument is concerned with *death*, not *the prospect of death*.

4. There is no doubt that the concept of experience plays a crucial role in the standard interpretation of the Epicurean argument. To understand the argument more clearly, I want to briefly illustrate what is meant by 'experience' in the standard interpretation of the Epicurean argument.

According to Rosenbaum (an Epicurean), there is an important supposition about experience used in the standard interpretation of the Epicurean argument: one can experience a state of affairs *only if* it can affect one in some way. In other words, according to Rosenbaum, there is *always* a causal element in experience. In this sense of 'experience', then, one does not experience a situation merely by believing that the situation has occurred or will occur, or by imagining a certain situation. With regard to this, Rosenbaum explicates:

> A person can believe that a state of affairs has occurred or will occur even if the state of affairs has had no causal effects on the person. The event may not have occurred and may never occur. Thus, in the sense of "experience" presupposed here, one does not experience just by believing. Similarly, one does not experience a situation just by imagining it. One might imagine oneself basking lazily on a sunny beach, but that situation is not thereby a situation that one experiences. The apparently required causal connection between the situation and the person is missing.[16]

He continues to explain:

> Notice that I have assumed here only a necessary condition for experiencing a situation, not a sufficient condition. Hence, one might be causally affected by a situation and not experience it. Perhaps awareness of the causal effects is also required. I believe there may

be one sense of the term "experience" in which awareness is required, another in which it is not. It is difficult to think that one could perceptually experience something, for example, without being aware of it. However, there is that way of experiencing in which we are said to undergo an experience, of which we need not be aware. If one undergoes (as we say) the experience of being irradiated by low level radioactivity, one might well not be aware of it. It seems to me that one clear requirement of experience, at least in one clear sense, is that one be causally affected in some way by situations one experiences.[17]

Anyhow, according to Rosenbaum, an essential requirement of experience is that one be causally affected in some way by the situation one experiences or undergoes.[18]

Basically, this view is acceptable. On the basis of this understanding, I now want to move on to make explicit the basic structure of the standard interpretation of the Epicurean argument.

First of all, (C)[19] is correct. This can be shown as follows:

> (1) Death is the permanent and irreversible cessation of one's existence (as assumed in Introduction).
> (2) Given (1), after P's death, there is *no subject*.
> (3) Given (2), after P's death, P cannot be causally affected in any way by any state of affairs.
> (4) One can experience a state of affairs *only if* it can affect one in some way.
> (5) Therefore, after P's death, P cannot experience any state of affairs.

The conclusion of this argument is logically equivalent to: P can experience a state of affairs *only if* he exists when the state of affairs obtains or occurs. This is clearly equivalent to (C)—P can experience a state of affairs only if it begins before P's death.

In the standard interpretation of the Epicurean argument, there are only three premises which are basic: (A), (C), and (D). The others, (B) and (E), are logical consequences of (A), (C), and (D). Since (D) is true by definition and (C) can be vindicated, as shown above, in order to reject the standard interpretation of the Epicurean argument, and thus, the Epicurean argument, the critical fire should be primarily concentrated on premise (A).

With the explication of the Epicurean argument concluded, we are now in a position to make a critique of the standard interpretation of the Epicurean argument, and thus, the Epicurean argument.

1.2 A CRITIQUE OF THE EPICUREAN ARGUMENT

It is evident that John's loss of his one leg in a car accident is a harm to him. He might suffer extreme discomfort and pains before, and indeed during, treatment. Besides this, he would lose the normal functioning of his leg, and, therefore, suffer inconvenience for the rest of his life. In addition to us considering this a harm, this would also be considered a harm according to the Epicurean position.

Most people believe that in most instances life is more important than a leg. That is to say, they believe that generally someone's death is a greater harm than losing a leg. When, for example, cutting off one leg is necessary for saving John's life, most people would judge that John should agree to the clinical amputation of his leg. However, according to the Epicurean argument, John's death by no means can be a harm to John. It sounds very odd. This suggests that something is seriously wrong with the Epicurean argument.

For the rest of this section, I want to demonstrate that the standard interpretation of the Epicurean argument (and thus, the Epicurean argument) is defective.

As shown in the last section, in order to reject the standard interpretation of the Epicurean argument, our attention should be primarily concentrated on premise (A)—a state of affairs (or event) is a harm (or bad thing) for someone P *only if* P can experience it. Let us therefore give (A) some more detailed consideration.

Put simply, the main point of the Epicurean argument is: Death cannot be a harm or misfortune for the person who dies, for, when death occurs, there is no longer a subject to whom any harm or misfortune can be ascribed.[20]

With this clear and straightforward interpretation, it can be seen that the Epicurean argument presupposes a principle—harm-requires-existence. This principle can be roughly understood as follows: *A requirement of a harm (or bad thing) for any person P is the existence of the subject P.* More explicitly, this principle is: Someone P can be the subject of some harm (or bad thing) *only if* he exists at the time the harm (or bad thing) occurs.[21] According to this principle, 'P exists when a state of affairs (or event) occurs' is a *necessary* condition for that state of affairs (or event) being a harm (or bad thing) for P. This means that if subject P does not exist when a state of affairs (or event) occurs, then that state of affairs (or event) cannot, and, thus, is not a harm (or bad thing) for P.

From this, it is reasonable to offer the following analysis of the Epicurean argument:

(1) If 'P exists when a state of affairs (or event) occurs' is merely a *necessary* (but not sufficient) condition for that state of affairs (or event) being a harm (or bad thing) for P, as the Epicurean argument assumes, then 'P exists when a state of affairs (or event) occurs' will not in itself bring it about that that state of affairs (or event) is a harm (or bad thing) for P. That is, in the Epicurean argument, 'P exists when a state of affairs (or event) occurs' is not the final reason (or essential factor) for the state of affairs (or event) being a harm (or bad thing) for P.

(2) However, according to the above analysis, the Epicurean argument assumes that if subject P does not exist when a state of affairs (or event) occurs, then that state of affairs (or event) cannot be a harm (or bad thing) for P.

(3) Given (1) and (2), the Epicurean argument implicitly asserts that '*P does not exist* when a state of affairs (or event) occurs' blocks or prevents any other more precise (or closer) necessary condition (or conditions) or even sufficient condition for that state of affairs (or event) being a harm (or bad thing) for P. In other words, in the Epicurean argument, Epicurus might well have supposed that there might be some other more precise necessary condition (or conditions) for a state of affairs (or event) being a harm (or bad thing) for P than 'P exists when that state of affairs (or event) occurs'.[22]

According to this analysis, the requirement for a more precise necessary condition for a state of affairs (or event) being a harm (or bad thing) for P would be: 'P exists when the state of affairs (or event) occurs' is a necessary condition for the more precise condition.

Now let us explore the more precise necessary condition in more detail.

The Epicurean argument presupposes that death is the total and permanent annihilation of consciousness.[23] Given this presupposition, it is impossible for someone P to experience anything after he dies. In other words, the Epicurean argument implicitly asserts that *only if* P exists when a state of affairs (or event) occurs, can P experience that state of affairs (or event). Accordingly, Epicurus should agree that 'P's not existing when a state of affairs (or event) occurs' blocks or rules out the possibility that P can experience that state of affairs (or event). That is to say, he should accept that 'P exists when a state of affairs (or event) occurs' is a necessary condition for 'P can experience the state of affairs (or event)'.

Furthermore, 'P can experience a state of affairs (or event)' could actually be accepted by Epicurus as a necessary condition for the state of affairs (or event) being a harm (or bad thing) for P. In the Epicurean argument, Epicurus claims, '...all good and evil consists in sensation...'[24] Sensation is a special kind of experience (or a part of experience). Thus, if P cannot experience anything, then P cannot and, therefore, does not, sense anything. This claim entails at least that experience is a necessary condition for 'all good and evil'. More explicitly, 'P can experience a state of affairs (or event)' is a necessary condition for the state of affairs (or event) being a good or an evil for P. Therefore, according to the Epicurean argument, a state of affairs (or event) is a harm (or bad thing) for someone P *only if* P can experience it. This is premise (A) in the standard interpretation of the Epicurean argument.

Accordingly, it is claimed that 'P can experience a state of affairs (or event)' is this more precise necessary condition for the state of affairs (or event) being a harm (or bad thing) for P.[25]

Given that, in the Epicurean argument 'P can experience a state of affairs (or event)' is a more precise (statement of a) necessary condition for the state of affairs (or event) being a harm (or bad thing) for P than 'P exists when a state of affairs (or event) occurs'[26], to claim that the Epicurean argument presupposes: 'A state of affairs (or event) is a harm (or bad thing) for someone P *only if* P can experience it' is more appropriate than to claim that the Epicurean argument presupposes: 'A state of affairs (or event) is a harm (or bad thing) for someone P *only if* P exists when it occurs'.

It is clear that the proposition 'If P cannot experience a state of affairs (or event), then it is not a harm (or bad thing) for P' (proposition (A*)) is logically equivalent to premise (A) in the standard interpretation of the Epicurean argument—a state of affairs (or event) is a harm (or bad thing) for someone P *only if* P can experience it. Rosenbaum (an Epicurean) offers an example (call this Case One) to support (A*), and, thus, (A):

Suppose that a person P *cannot* hear and never will hear. Then the egregious performance of a Mozart symphony *cannot* causally affect P at any time, supposing that what makes the performance bad is merely awful sound, detectable only through normal hearing, and supposing further that the performance does not initiate uncommon causal sequences that can affect the person. It is clear that the person *cannot* experience the bad performance, auditorily or otherwise...It *cannot* affect the person in any way. The reason why it is not bad for him is that he *is not able to* experience it. The person's being deaf insulates him from auditory experiences that might otherwise be bad for him. Similarly, a person born without a sense of smell *cannot* be causally affected by, and thus *cannot* experience, the stench of a smouldering cheroot. The stench *cannot* be an olfactory negativity for her. We could imagine indefinitely many more such cases...Dead persons *cannot* experience any state of affairs; they are blind, deaf, and generally insentient.[27] (My emphasis.)

Before discussing Case One, it is very important to briefly make explicit the compound concept 'P *cannot* experience a (particular) state of affairs (or event)' in Case One, and, thus, (A*). The compound concept 'P *cannot* experience a (particular) state of affairs (or event)' is ambiguous. It can express at least three different kinds of impossibility of P's experiencing a (particular) state of affairs (or event):

(1) Logical or metaphysical: The impossibility of P's experiencing a (particular) state of affairs (or event) may be logical or metaphysical. In other words, P cannot experience a (particular) state of affairs (or event), because the supposed state of affairs (or event) (or the experience of it) is, conceptually, *contradictory* or *impossible*. For example, P cannot experience at the same time 'eating an apple' and 'not eating an apple'. Or it is impossible for P to swim and not to swim in Brisbane River at the same time.

(2) Physical: The impossibility of P's experiencing a (particular) state of affairs (or event) may be physical. In other words, P cannot experience a (particular) state of affairs (or event), because the supposed state of affairs (or event) (or the experience of it) conflicts with laws of nature. In this case, the supposed state of affairs (or event) can be logically or metaphysically possible (i.e. it can be conceptually consistent or possible). For example, P

cannot experience 'floating in the air without any support'. Or it is impossible for P to experience 'sitting in a space shuttle whose velocity is faster than the velocity of light'.

(3) Situational (or practical): The impossibility of P's experiencing a (particular) state of affairs (or event) may be situational (or practical). In other words, P cannot experience a (particular) state of affairs (or event), because the supposed state of affairs (or event) is not genuinely open, accessible, or realisable by P. For example, it is impossible for an untrained and overweight athlete to win an Olympic gold medal.[28]

Clearly, 'P cannot *logically* or *metaphysically* experience a (particular) state of affairs (or event)' entails 'P cannot *physically* experience the state of affairs (or event)'. A state of affairs (or event) may be *physically* possible but impossible nevertheless in this situational (or practical) sense.

Now, the question here is: What does the statement 'P cannot experience a (particular) state of affairs (or event)' in Case One, and, thus, (A*) mean? Is it (1), (2), (3) or something else? I suggest that (1) is the appropriate answer. The reason is as follows. In Case One, during all his life, P completely lacks his sense of, for example, hearing. It is conceptually impossible that P hears the performance. Thus, P, in Case One, is logically or metaphysically unable (without any special prosthetic) to hear this performance.

If we give Case One our very careful consideration, however, we will find a more precise reason why the performance is not bad for P which is not that 'he is not [metaphysically] able to experience it' as Rosenbaum claims. I suggest that the reason can be: He *does not* experience it. To show this, let us consider another two cases which are modified from Case One:

> Case Two. The facts are the same as in Case One, except that Q, who can hear properly, goes to the concert to listen to this performance with P. Before the performance starts, Q feels uncomfortable and goes to the toilet. After he leaves the toilet, the performance has finished. Q never has any knowledge about this performance.

> Case Three. Suppose R can smell properly. When his flatmate smokes a foul cheroot in their flat, he goes outside for his lunch.

Suppose we take the Epicurean view, and thus maintain, as Rosenbaum claims in Case One, that the performance is not a bad thing for P because he is not (logically or metaphysically) able to experience it. (Note that, in this case, 'P is logically or metaphysically able to experience the performance' is a *necessary* condition for the performance being a bad thing for him.) In considering Case Two, it would be reasonable for us to judge that the performance is not a bad thing for Q either. After all, Q *does not* experience the performance. Similarly, in Case Three, it would be very strange for us to believe that the foul smell is a bad thing for R. After all, R *does not* experience the foul smell.

All of this suggests that if Epicureans (including Rosenbaum, and, of course, Epicurus) intend to make their view more reasonable, more systematic, and more consistent, then they should concede that 'P experiences a state of affairs (or event) when that state of affairs (or event) occurs' is also a *necessary* condition for the state of affairs (or event) being a harm (or bad thing) for P.

So far, I have shown that in the Epicurean argument it has been assumed that 'P can experience a state of affairs (or event)' is a necessary condition for the state of affairs (or event) being a harm (or bad thing) for P. Again, since 'P can experience a state of affairs (or event)' is merely a *necessary* (but not a sufficient) condition for the state of affairs (or event) being a harm (or bad thing) for P, it is reasonable for us to suppose that in the Epicurean argument, some other more precise necessary (or even a sufficient) condition for a state of affairs (or event) being a harm (or bad thing) for P has been assumed than 'P can experience the state of affairs (or event)'. The requirement for this more precise necessary condition, according to the above analysis, would be: 'P can experience a state of affairs (or event)' is a necessary condition for this more precise condition.

Apparently, as was shown above, 'P experiences a state of affairs (or event) when that state of affairs (or event) occurs' can meet this requirement. Therefore, 'P experiences a state of affairs (or event) when that state of affairs (or event) occurs' would be this more precise necessary condition for the state of affairs (or event) being a harm (or bad thing) for P. This means that the reason that 'P can experience a state of affairs (or event)' is a necessary condition for the state of affairs (or event) being a harm (or bad thing) for P is based on the supposition that 'P experiences a state of affairs (or event) when that state of affairs (or event) occurs' is a necessary condition for the state of affairs (or event) being a harm (or bad thing) for P. In other words, premise (A) in the standard interpretation of the Epicurean argument can be derived from the supposition that 'P experiences a state of affairs (or event) when that state of affairs (or event) occurs' is a necessary condition for the state of affairs (or event) being a harm (or bad thing) for P.

Now the next question to be addressed is: What does the Epicurean argument assume as the *sufficient* condition for a state of affairs (or event) being a harm (or bad thing) for P?

To answer this question, let us look back to Case Two and Case Three.

Suppose we take the Epicurean view and believe that the performance is not a bad thing for P because he *does not* experience it. Suppose also that in Case Two, Q has listened to the performance. However, suppose that Q feels excited by the unusual sound, and, thus, does not treat the performance as *egregious*. In this circumstance, it would be very strange for us to claim that the performance is a bad thing for Q. Conversely, it is reasonable for us to claim that if Q experiences the performance and feels it as bad, then the performance is a bad thing for him. On the other hand, we would claim that if Q experiences the performance and feels it as good, then the performance is a good thing for him.

Similarly, suppose in Case Three R has smelt the smouldering cheroot. However, suppose he really enjoys this kind of smell. In this circumstance, we would not think that the smouldering cheroot is a bad thing for R. Conversely, we are inclined to think that if R experiences the smouldering cheroot and feels it as bad, then the smouldering cheroot is a bad thing for him. On the other hand, it is natural for us to think that if R experiences the smouldering cheroot and feels it as good, then the smouldering cheroot is a good thing for him.

All of this suggests that if Epicureans (including Epicurus, of course) want to make their view more reasonable, more systematic, and more consistent, then they should assert that 'P experiences a state of affairs (or event) when that state of affairs (or event) occurs' is not a *sufficient* condition for the state of affairs (or event) being a harm (or bad thing) for P. The *sufficient* condition for the state of affairs (or event) being a harm (or bad thing) for P would be: P experiences *and feels the state of affairs (or event) as bad* when the state of affairs (or event) occurs.[29]

So far, we have identified what is, in the Epicurean argument, the final reason (or *essential* factor) for a state of affairs (or event) being a harm (or bad thing) for P. And this means that the reason for 'P experiences a state of affairs (or event) when that state of affairs (or event) occurs' to be a *necessary* condition for the state of affairs (or event) being a harm (or bad thing) for P is based on this *sufficient* condition—P experiences *and feels the state of affairs (or event) as bad* when the state of affairs (or event) occurs.

To sum up, according to the above discussion about premise (A) in the standard interpretation of the Epicurean argument, the Epicurean argument has made four assumptions:

> (1) 'P exists when a state of affairs (or event) occurs' is a necessary condition for the state of affairs (or event) being a harm (or bad thing) for P.
> (2) 'P can (logically or metaphysically) experience a state of affairs (or event)' is a more precise necessary condition for the state of affairs (or event) being a harm (or bad thing) for P.
> (3) 'P experiences a state of affairs (or event) when the state of affairs (or event) occurs' is a much more precise necessary condition for the state of affairs (or event) being a harm (or bad thing) for P.
> (4) 'P experiences and feels a state of affairs (or event) as bad when the state of affairs (or event) occurs' is a *sufficient* condition for the state of affairs (or event) being a harm (or bad thing) for P. 'P experiences and feels a state of affairs (or event) as good when the state of affairs (or event) occurs' is a *sufficient* condition for the state of affairs (or event) being a good thing for P.[30]

Now we are in a good position to reject premise (A) in the standard interpretation of Epicurean argument, and, thus, this construal of the Epicurean argument.

To reject the former part of (4)—'P experiences and feels a state of affairs (or event) as bad when the state of affairs (or event) occurs' is a *sufficient* condition for the state of affairs (or event) being a harm (or bad thing) for P—let us consider the following example:

> Case Four. Suppose someone P is infected with an unknown virus. This virus will change his gene structure and reduce his life by 10 years. Moreover, all his offspring will inherit the bad gene and have 10 fewer years to live. This disease will not cause any pain or affect any normal life. Now, there is a new medicinal product which can completely cure this disease. This product is very safe. Since P hates injections, he is forcibly taken to the hospital to be given an injection by his parents. As a result, he experiences pain, and feels a little bit

uncomfortable from side effects. Afterwards, he refuses to go to the hospital again.

Before discussing this case, it is very important to distinguish (i) the overall value of a state of affairs (or event), from (ii) a partial value of a state of affairs (or event). If a state of affairs (or event) can be evaluated in different respects, then the evaluation of that state of affairs (or event) in each respect yields a partial value. On the other hand, if we evaluate the state of affairs (or event) for all its partial values, then this (final) evaluation is its overall value. Apparently, if a state of affairs (or event) can be evaluated in only one respect, then this evaluation will determine the overall value.

According to the former part of (4), it would be claimed that, in Case Four, the injection is bad for P. For P *does* experience and feel discomfort from this injection. However, this injection will prevent misfortune later—less life for him and his offspring. Thus, it is reasonable for us to judge that, in Case Four, overall this injection is good for him. Of course, the pain and discomfort from the injection is a bad thing for P. However, this bad thing is only one of the partial values of this injection, not an overall one. In fact, in Case Four, there is still some other partial value of this injection which is good for P. It is because of this other partial value of this injection that we judge this injection to be good *overall* for P. According to this analysis, it is problematic to claim that ˙P experiences and feels a state of affairs (or event) as bad when the state of affairs (or event) occurs˙ is a *sufficient* condition for the state of affairs (or event) being *overall* a bad thing for P (though it can be a *partial* bad thing for P). In short, the former part of (4) is compromised.

As to the latter part of (4)—˙P experiences and feels a state of affairs (or event) as good when the state of affairs (or event) occurs˙ is a *sufficient* condition for the state of affairs (or event) being a good thing for P—Nagel offers a good example (which I shall call Case Five) to refute this:

> Suppose an intelligent person receives a brain injury that reduces him to the mental condition of a contented infant, and that such desires as remain to him can be satisfied by a custodian, so that he is free from care. Such a development would be widely regarded as a severe misfortune, not only for his friends and relations, or for society, but also, and primarily, for the person himself.[31]

In Case Five, suppose this person took a pride in his intelligence before his brain injury. In addition, suppose he did not always feel very happy because of his high self-esteem. Suppose also he does not suffer any pain during the process of his brain injury. Suppose, besides, he feels very happy and satisfied all the time after his brain injury. According to the latter part of (4), in Case Five, the state of affairs this person is in now would be a good thing for him, since he *experiences and feels* the state of affairs as good. However, this is totally counterintuitive and unacceptable. To show the unreasonability of the latter part of (4), let us consider another, even clearer, example:

> Case Six. Someone P is fed a drug by Q when he is sleeping. The process does not cause P any discomfort. After that, P is taken away to Q's place. Q treats P as a slave and often abuses him. Because the drug makes P enjoy what Q does to him, P likes to be Q's slave.[32]

Do you, after considering this case, think: 'What a wonderful life Q is leading now. I wish I, or my children, could lead it'? Can we, following the latter part of (4), claim that, in Case Six the state P is in now is a good thing for P? Surely not! In this case, Q at least loses his psychological freedom. Moreover, his dignity is badly damaged. In short, we judge this to be a harm because we recognise that it is a state that we would prefer not be in. This shows that we can be harmed even though we are unable to know (i.e. recognise) that we are harmed.

I have shown that the Epicurean argument presupposes (4). Since both parts of (4) are problematic, the Epicurean argument is problematic.

To my criticism, Epicureans might reply:

> The Epicurean argument does not presuppose (4). That is a misunderstanding of the Epicurean argument. What it really presupposes is only (3)—'P experiences a state of affairs (or event) when the state of affairs (or event) occurs' is a *necessary* condition for the state of affairs (or event) being a harm (or bad thing) for P.

Even though Epicureans maybe right at this point, (3) is still incorrect. Consider the following case:

> Case Seven. Suppose a person P had a lovely family—with a beautiful and sweet wife, a clever and cute son, and a friendly dog. P was a good man and had a very good reputation which he was very proud of. Q was P's good friend. Two years ago, P went to an island

to do some business for six months. After he left for this island, Q started trying to convince P's wife and son that P actually was an evil man. Unbelievably, they had fallen for the malicious lies of Q and come to hate P. Sadly, from that time on, P's wife had an affair with Q. Q also passed vile, false rumours to all P's friends to damage P's reputation. All P's friends believed Q's lies. P was completely unaware of this. When he came back, he still lived with his family and still treated Q as a good friend. And also he was still very proud of his 'good' reputation. However, P did not suffer as a result.[33]

In Case Seven, although P does not actually *experience* this misfortune, we would judge that he was severely harmed by this event. It is very clear that he lost at least his reputation and the loyalty of his wife. And both the reputation and the loyalty of his wife are in his interests. He might have done everything he could to secure (or enhance) them. Anyhow, his interests were seriously frustrated in this event. That is, he was badly harmed (at least in a sense). However, according to (3), P was not harmed by this event.

I grant that it might be more harmful if P knew (experienced) all of this. However, this should not be considered support for the claim that what you do not know (or experience) cannot hurt you. There is still room for the unexperienced harms in addition to the experienced ones (this will be discussed in Chapter Four). Indeed, as George Pitcher correctly points out :

> ...it is just false that in order to be harmed, the victim must be aware of the harm. To be sure, in most cases of misfortune, the victim is aware of the (for him) unfortunate state of affairs. But a misfortune can befall a person who is totally ignorant of it.[34]

In some cases, one might believe that what he loses is more important regardless of whether or not he knows it (or even how he feels). Suppose a powerful and malicious killer tells me (and I do have reason to believe) he will destroy all the people in New York City (including my wife and daughters) unless I take a special drug. The special drug will make me believe that they have all been killed. In such a case, I would agree to the deal as long as their safety is ensured.[35]

Accordingly, (3) is incorrect. As Epicureans grant, the Epicurean argument presupposes (3). Since (3) is incorrect, the Epicurean argument must be rejected.

To this, a defender of Epicureans might reply:

The Epicurean argument does not presuppose (3). According to the Epicurean argument, what we can grant is *merely* that: the Epicurean argument presupposes that 'P exists when a state of affairs (or event) occurs' is a *necessary* condition for the state of affairs (or event) being a harm (or bad thing) for P.

According to this reply, Epicureans concede that, in Case Seven P was harmed by this event. That is, the (existence) presupposition is logically consistent with the claim that P was harmed in Case Seven. However, they still insist that if P was dead when the event occurred, then this event would not be a harm to him.

Unfortunately, this (existence) presupposition is problematic as well. Let us consider the following case (call it Case Eight) raised by McMahan:

> ...consider the case of a person on holiday on a remote island. Back home, on Friday, his life's work collapses. But, because of the inaccessibility of the island, the bad news does not arrive until the following Monday. On the intervening Sunday, however, the man is killed by a shark; so he never learns that his life's work has come to nothing.[36]

As argued above, Epicureans should agree that, in Case Eight, the fact that his life's work has come to nothing is a harm or misfortune for him. McMahan offers the following reason to refute this (existence) presupposition:

> On reflection, it seems hard to believe that it makes a difference to the [harm or] misfortune he suffers whether the collapse of his life's work occurs shortly before he is killed or shortly afterward. Yet, according to the Existence Requirement [this presupposition], this difference in timing make *all* the difference. If the collapse of his life's work occurs just before he dies, then, even though he never learns of it, he suffers a terrible [harm or] misfortune. If, on the other hand, it occurs just after he dies, he suffers no [harm or] misfortune at all. If we find this hard to believe then we maybe forced to reject the Existence Requirement [this presupposition].[37]

Accordingly, this (existence) presupposition should be rejected. As Epicureans grant, the Epicurean argument presupposes that 'P exists when a state of affairs (or event) occurs' is a *necessary* condition for the state of affairs (or event) being a harm (or bad thing) for P. Since this (existence) presupposition is incorrect, the Epicurean argument is incorrect as well.[38]

The Epicurean argument concludes that death is *never* a harm to the person who dies. Since I have shown that the Epicurean argument is incorrect, at least I can confidently claim that thus far it is possible that death *can* be a harm to the person who dies. However, to reach this conclusion—death can actually be a harm to the person who dies—further argument is needed.

There are main two theories which try to justify or explain the harm of death: the desire-thwarting theory and the deprivation theory. I will proceed to discus these two theories in Chapter Two and Chapter Three respectively.

CHAPTER TWO

The Desire-thwarting Theory

This chapter is concerned with the questions: Is the desire-thwarting theory acceptable? If not, why? Let me outline this theory first.

Most philosophers cannot accept the conclusion of the Epicurean argument. In order to reject it, some of them have adopted the desire-thwarting (or desire-frustration) theory. This theory is based on a principle that *something is a harm or misfortune for us if it thwarts our desires; or something is a harm or misfortune for us if it thwarts the fulfilment of our desires.*[1] Speaking roughly, the desire-thwarting theory can be expressed by the following argument:

> (1) Something is a harm or misfortune for us if it thwarts our desires.
> (2) Death thwarts our desires.
> (3) Therefore, death is a harm or misfortune for us.[2]

Call this argument the 'original argument'.

The desire-thwarting theory is defended, most notably, by Bernard Williams. Let me now briefly outline Williams' defence of the desire-thwarting theory.

In his admirable paper "The Makropulos Case: Reflections on the Tedium of Immortality", Williams argues:

> If I desire something, then, other things being equal, I prefer a state of affairs in which I get it from one in which I do not get it, and (again, other things being equal) plan for a future in which I get it rather than not. But one future, for sure, in which I would not get it would be one in which I was dead. To want something, we may also say, is to that extent to have reason for resisting what excludes having that thing: and death certainly does that, for a very large range of things that one wants. If that is right, then for any of those things, wanting something itself gives one a reason for avoiding death. Even though if I do not succeed, I will not know that, nor what I am missing, from the perspective of the wanting agent it is rational to aim for states of affairs in which his want is satisfied, and hence to regard death as something to be avoided; that is, to regard it as an evil.[3]

If Williams' exploration of the desire-thwarting theory goes only as far as this stage, then perhaps his desire-thwarting theory can be expressed by the original argument. However, his account does not end here. He continues to elucidate it by distinguishing between 'conditional' and 'unconditional' (or categorical) desires.[4]

Conditional desires can be understood as desires about a situation at some future time which depend on the assumption that we shall be alive at that time; if we think that we shall be dead, we are indifferent about the situation.[5] Williams gives the following explanation of conditional desires:

> It is admittedly true that many of the things I want, I want only on the assumption that I am going to be alive; and some people, for instance some of the old, desperately want certain things when nevertheless they would much rather that they and their wants were dead.[6]

Fischer also offers an easy and clear example: 'For example, one might want to be treated well, if one remains alive, but wish, all things considered, that one were dead.'[7]

More formally, conditional desires can be put in the following way:

> I want the following to be the case: If I am alive at T, then X will be the case at T (X is some state of affairs or situation which my conditional desire concerns).[8]

On the other hand, desires that are not in this way dependent on our being alive are *unconditional*.

It is very clear, on this analysis, and as Williams also believes, that death cannot thwart conditional desires. However, Williams believes that death *can* thwart unconditional (categorical) desires. Therefore, he claims that death's harm consists in its frustration of a person's unconditional (or categorical) desires.[9] This is a brief outline of Williams' defence of the desire-thwarting theory.

According to the above discussion, it is obvious that the original argument is flawed. Thus, it is not suitable to use the original argument to defend the desire-thwarting theory. For Williams the original argument should be modified as:

> (1) Something is a harm or misfortune for us if it thwarts any of our desires.
> (2) Death thwarts our *unconditional* (or categorical) desires.
> (3) Therefore, death is a harm or misfortune for us.

Call this argument the 'unconditional argument'.

In other words, the desire-thwarting theory, for Williams, should be expressed by the unconditional argument.

It is clear that theoretically the unconditional argument is more appropriate than the original argument. However, Steven Luper-Foy rejects the unconditional argument. Luper-Foy believes that *not all* unconditional desires can be thwarted by death. Indeed, there are some unconditional desires which cannot be thwarted by death. To show this, he distinguishes 'dependent' and 'independent' desires.

With regard to independent desires, he says:

> Some of our aims [or desires] are such that our chances of
> successfully accomplishing them are not really affected by what we
> do in the course of our lives or even by whether or not we are alive.
> Being alive does not help us achieve these ends [or desires]; hence
> they cannot be thwarted by our deaths...call these *independent* goals
> [or desires]...My desire that the moon continue to orbit Earth, for
> example, is an independent goal [or desire]...[10]

On the other hand, dependent desires are expressed by Luper-Foy as, '[Those
goals or desires] whose chances of being achieved do depend on our activities
we can call *dependent* goals [or desires].'[11]

In short, asserts Luper-Foy, there can be two kinds of unconditional
desires—independent unconditional desires and dependent unconditional
desires. Although dependent unconditional desires can be thwarted by death,
independent unconditional desires cannot.

Fischer also makes a similar point. He distinguishes the following two
kinds of 'unconditional (or categorical)' desires:

(1) Impersonal unconditional desires: desires that some condition
obtain in the future irrespective of its causal genesis. For
example, we want it to be the case that poverty, starvation, and
disease are eradicated, that political oppression is ended, that
our environment is preserved, that our families, friends, and
nations prosper, and so on.

(2) Egocentric unconditional desires: desires that some condition
obtain in the future as a result of what I do. For example, I may
wish not just that a book is written, but that a book is written *by
me*, and I may wish not just that a family is raised, but that a
family is raised *by me*, and so forth.[12]

Obviously, at least in certain contexts, 'impersonal unconditional' desires
cannot be thwarted by death.

Accordingly, it is apparent that the unconditional argument is defective or
at least needs modification. Thus, it is not suitable to use the unconditional

argument to express the desire-thwarting theory. For Luper-Foy, the unconditional argument should be modified as:

> (1) Something is a harm or misfortune for us if it thwarts any of our desires.
> (2) Death thwarts *certain* kind(s) of our unconditional desires.
> (3) Therefore, death is a harm or misfortune for us.

Call this argument the 'desire-thwarting argument'.

In other words, the desire-thwarting theory, for Luper-Foy, should be expressed by the desire-thwarting argument. Apparently, the desire-thwarting argument is theoretically more satisfactory than the unconditional argument.

So understood, the desire-thwarting theory seems very reasonable. However, in the next section, I will show that even the desire-thwarting theory is expressed by the desire-thwarting argument—the best version of the three—it is still problematic.

2.2 SHORTCOMINGS OF THE DESIRE-THWARTING THEORY

According to the analysis in the last section, the desire-thwarting theory can be appropriately expressed as:

> (1) Something is a harm or misfortune for us if it thwarts any of our desires.
> (2) Death thwarts *certain* kind(s) of our unconditional desires.
> (3) Therefore, death is a harm or misfortune for us.

Call this argument the 'desire-thwarting argument'.

Unfortunately, the desire-thwarting argument, and, thus, the desire-thwarting theory, is flawed. Let me now demonstrate the reason.

In the desire-thwarting argument, (3) is a logical consequence of (1) and (2). (2) can be generally accepted.[13] Thus, if the desire-thwarting argument is problematic, then the essential problem should be in (1). In other words, in order to reject the desire-thwarting argument, and, thus, the desire-thwarting theory, the focus should be entirely located on premise (1) in the desire-thwarting argument.

Let us now examine premise (1) in the desire-thwarting argument in more detail.

In his paper "Harm to Others", Joel Feinberg distinguishes a pair of conceptions:

> (1) Want-fulfilment: the coming into existence of that which is desired.
> (2) Want-satisfaction: the pleasant experience of contentment or gratification that normally occurs in the mind of the desirer when he believes that his desire has been fulfilled.[14]

Feinberg explicates this distinction as follows:

> When the object of a want does not come into existence, we can say that the want has been *unfulfilled* or *thwarted*; the experience in the mind of the desirer when he believes that his desire has been thwarted is called frustration or disappointment.[15]

Here, Feinberg emphasises that the occurrence of subjective satisfaction is a highly unreliable indicator of fulfilment. He says:

> Sometimes when our goals are achieved, we do not experience much joy, but only fatigue and sadness, or an affective blankness. Some persons, perhaps, are disposed by temperament normally to receive their achievements in this unthrilled fashion...Not only can one have fulfilment without satisfaction; one can also have satisfaction of a want in the absence of its actual fulfilment, provided only that one is led to believe, falsely, that one's want has been fulfilled.[16]

On the other hand, Feinberg asserts that this highly contingent and unreliable phenomenon occurs in the case of one's subjective disappointment as well. He writes:

...one's wants can be thwarted without causing frustration, or disappointment, and one can be quite discontented even when one's wants have in fact been fulfilled...A perfectly genuine and well-considered goal may be thwarted without causing mental pain when the desirer has a placid temperament or a stoic philosophy. And discontent does not presuppose thwarting of desire any more than satisfaction presupposes fulfilment. One can have feelings of frustration and disappointment caused by false beliefs that one's wants have been thwarted, or by drugs and other manipulative techniques.[17]

Accordingly, Feinberg concludes that harm is best defined in terms of the *objective thwarting of desires* rather than in subjective terms.[18] In other words, for Feinberg, harm would be defined as something which thwarts the *fulfilment* of our desires. Apparently, this is (1) in the desire-thwarting argument. In short, Feinberg endorses (1).

Feinberg also gives the following reasons to support this conclusion:

(i) Most people will agree that the important thing is to get what they want, even if that causes no joy.

(ii) The pleasure that normally attends want-fulfilment is a welcome dividend, but the object of our efforts is to fulfil our wants in the world, not to bring about subjective states of our own minds.

(iii) If (ii) were not the case, there would be no way to account for the pleasure of satisfaction when it does come; we are satisfied only because we think that our desires are fulfilled. In other words, if the object of our desires were valuable to us only as a means to our inner states of pleasure, those glows could never come.[19]

It may be that Feinberg has here successfully shown:

(i) Want-nonfulfilment and want-disappointment are different conceptions. It is not necessary for them to be jointly satisfied; and

(ii) It is not appropriate to define harm in terms of the subjective disappointment of desires (wants), because subjective disappointments (and satisfactions) are highly contingent and unreliable phenomena.

However, Feinberg does not offer enough reasons for the conclusion that harm is best defined in terms of the objective nonfulfilment of desires (wants). In other words, he does not give sufficient reasons to support (1) in the desire-thwarting argument. Indeed, (1) is problematic. The reason is simply that it is not correct that whatever thwarts one's desires is a harm or misfortune for one. This can be shown as follows.

First of all, quite a lot of our desires, perhaps even most of them, are very trivial. For example:

> I desire to drink some water five minutes later in my office, provided that the failure to do so would not lead to any health problem or any possible harm (e.g. social harm). And I can easily get some soda water or coke drink in my office.

> or

> I hope tomorrow's weather will be good enough for me to see the bright moon with my girlfriend. However, if the weather is bad, I can still listen to my favourite classical music with her.

It is not apparent whether or not the nonfulfilment of my desires in these cases can be counted as a *harm* to me. It seems odd to treat it as a *harm* to me. After all, the desires here are too trivial. Unless acceptable reasons have been given, it is questionable to see the thwarting of our trivial desires as a harm to us. (I do not want to discuss this issue any further here.)

Even if the thwarting of these trivial desires could reasonably be treated as a harm, we can still have at least the following four kinds of desires (which may be trivial or more important) whose nonfulfilment would not be appropriately counted as a harm to us.

(I). *Anti-logical Desires.* Desires can be arbitrarily formed. In theory, we can desire anything. Indeed, as Derek Parfit points out, we can desire (want) something to be true even when we know that it is logically impossible for this desire to be fulfilled. For example, 'The Pythagoreans wanted [desired] the square root of two to be a rational number.'[20]

It would be very strange to insist that the nonfulfilment of our anti-logical desires is a harm to us. At most, perhaps, it is source of a regret for us.

(II). *Anti-physical Desires.* We might occasionally desire something which is contrary to the physical theories. For instance, we might want (desire) to float in the sky or walk on the water without any special equipment.

There is no doubt that the nonfulfilment of our anti-physical desires cannot reasonably be regarded as a harm to us either.

(III). *Highly Improbable Desires.* We might also, once in a while, desire something which, although logically and physically possible, is highly improbable. For instance, someone P desires to be the president of the USA the next week. This amounts to a *practical* impossibility in the sense outlined in Chapter One.

Suppose P's desire is thwarted. Yet, it is not proper to think that P has been harmed.

(IV). *Harmful Desires.* Furthermore, we can even have desires whose fulfilment is a harm to us. Rosenbaum offers the following example:

> Suppose that a person for some reason desires to avoid being vaccinated against various diseases to which the person could succumb if not vaccinated—polio, smallpox, typhoid fever, or others.[21]

Apparently, thwarting this desire would be good for the person, for it would reduce the likelihood of suffering later. In short, as Rosenbaum says, some desires persons have would not be good to fulfil, and it would be good for those persons that those desires be thwarted.[22]

These four kinds of desires would constitute some proportion of our desires. Thus, since these are desires whose nonfulfilment is not a harm, (1) in the desire-thwarting argument—Something is a harm or misfortune for us *if* it thwarts our desires—is mistaken and the desire-thwarting argument as presented in Chapter Two, Section One is unsound.

However, although the desire-thwarting theory is at least problematic, this does not mean that the conclusion of the desire-thwarting argument—death is a harm or misfortune for us—is incorrect. Indeed, from the above discussion, the main conclusion to draw is merely: The desire-thwarting theory cannot justify the claim that death is a harm or misfortune for us. It may still be the case that death is a harm or misfortune for us. To show why death is a harm or misfortune for us, we need to find some other argument or theory, or at least to modify the desire-thwarting account.

Given this, the alternative theory—the deprivation theory—might provide an account of the badness of death. Let us now move on to the deprivation theory.

CHAPTER THREE

The Deprivation Theory

The deprivation theory is the most popular anti-Epicurean view.[1] Silverstein calls this view the standard argument against the Epicurean view.[2] In this chapter, I want to investigate whether or not this very popular anti-Epicurean view is satisfactory. To begin this task, let me first illustrate the deprivation theory.

In his well-known paper "Death", Nagel claims, 'If death is an evil at all, it cannot be because of its positive features, but only because of what it deprives us of.'[3]

Basically, this claim has pointed to a rough and vague picture of the deprivation theory. Nagel explicates the deprivation theory as follows:

> ...if death is an evil, it is the loss of life, rather than the state of being dead, or nonexistent, or unconscious, that is objectionable...
>
> If we are to make sense of the view that to die is bad, it must be on the ground that life is a good and death is the *corresponding deprivation or loss*, bad not because of any positive features but because of the desirability of what it removes.[4] (My emphasis.)

Similarly, Williams says:

[The Epicurean view] takes it as genuinely true of life that the satisfaction of desire, and possession of the *praemia vitae*, are good things...But now if we consider two lives, one very short and cut off before the *praemia* have been acquired, the other fully provided with the *praemia* and containing their enjoyment to a ripe age, it is very difficult to see why the second life, by these standards alone, is not to be thought better than the first...But if the *praemia vitae* are valuable...then surely getting to the point of possessing them is better than not getting to that point, longer enjoyment of them is better than shorter, and more of them, other things being equal, is better than less of them. But if so, then it just will not be true...that death is never an evil...[5]

Also, L. W. Sumner says:

To die is (as we say) to lose one's life. Generally speaking, a loss is a bad thing to the extent that the item lost is a good thing...Losing one's life must therefore be an evil when, and to the extent that, one's life is a good. Let us be more precise. Suppose that I own a fine watch for a year and then mislay it. What precisely have I lost? I cannot lose the year's possession and use of the watch, for that is in the past. What I have lost, then, is the use of the watch which I would have enjoyed had I continued to possess it. Losses are *future-oriented*: the main source of evil of a loss is the value which is thereby *foregone*...

We may therefore consider the misfortune of death as a loss and calculate its evil principally in terms of the value which it forecloses.[6] (My emphasis.)

In summary, the deprivation theory can be explicated as follows: *Death is a harm to the person who dies because it deprives him of certain goods—the goods he would have enjoyed if he had not died.*

According to the deprivation theory, death is simply the harm of deprivation, a harm consisting in the loss, or lack, of possible *future* goods.[8] Basically, the deprivation theorists believe that death is the unequivocal and permanent end of life and thus, an experiential blank.[9] Thus, death, for them, is not a peculiarly terrifying state that one somehow exists to suffer from.

In the face of this account, it is natural for some people (especially Epicureans) to wonder:

How can death be a harm to the person who dies, if it is *merely* an experiential blank? In other words, can anything, which is not actually experienced as bad or unpleasant by a person, be a harm to him?

To defend and strengthen their theory, the deprivation theorists need at least to justify the following principle: Something that is never actually experienced as bad or unpleasant by a person *can* be a harm to him. Indeed, Nagel argues for this principle as follows:

> We must now turn to the serious difficulties...about loss and privation in general, and about death in particular.
>
> Essentially, there are three types of problems. First, doubt may be raised whether *anything* can be bad for a man without being positively unpleasant to him: specifically, it may be doubted that there are any evils that consist merely in the deprivation or absence of possible goods...
>
> The first type of objection is expressed in general form by the common remark that what you don't know can't hurt you. It means that even if a man is betrayed by his friends, ridiculed behind his back, and despised by people who treat him politely to his face, none of it can be counted as a misfortune for him so long as he does not suffer as a result. It means that a man is not injured if his wishes are ignored by the executor of his will, or if, after his death, the belief becomes current that all the literary works on which his fame rests were really written by his brother, who died in Mexico at the age of 28...
>
> There certainly are goods and evils of a simple kind (including some pleasures and pains) which a person possesses at a given time simply in virtue of his condition at that time. But this is not true of all the things we regard as good or bad for a man...[10]

Similarly, Robert Nozick says:

> ...suppose we read the biography of a man who *felt* happy, took pride in his work, family life, etc. But we also read that his children, secretly, despised him; his wife, secretly, scorned him having innumerable affairs; his work was a subject of ridicule among all others, who kept their opinion from him; *every* source of satisfaction

in this man's life was built upon a falsehood, a deception. Do you, in reading about this man's life, think: 'What a *wonderful* life. I wish I, or my children, could lead it'?[11]

I think that the examples in these two arguments have successfully justified this principle. Given this principle, some proponents of the deprivation theory might incautiously conclude that death *can* be a harm to the person who dies, even if it is a *mere* experiential blank.

However, some opponents of the deprivation theory, such as Rosenbaum, try to reject the deprivation theory by arguing as follows:

> We agree that certain things never actually experienced as unpleasant or bad by a person can be a harm to that person. However, we cannot agree with the claim that death can be a harm to the person who dies. It is believed that the only way something can be a harm to a person is if it is *possible* for the person to experience it as unpleasant or bad. In other words, someone *can* be the subject of some harm *only if* he exists at the time the harm occurs—the Existence Requirement. But death—being an experiential blank that occurs after the person is alive or exists—cannot be experienced by the person who dies as unpleasant or bad. Thus, death cannot be a harm to the person who dies. Now the proponents of the deprivation theory adduce examples in which it is allegedly true that persons suffer harms or misfortunes of which they are unaware. But since none of these examples is an example in which the person has ceased to exist, and thus it is *impossible* for that person to experience the things as unpleasant or bad, none of the examples refutes the Existence Requirement. Thus, death should not be a harm to the person who dies [12]

This argument can be expressed as follows:

> (1) If the Existence Requirement is accepted, then this principle—something that is never actually experienced as bad or unpleasant by a person *can* be a harm to him—*cannot* apply to death. That is, if the Existence Requirement is accepted, then death *cannot* be a harm to the person who dies.
>
> (2) If death *cannot* be a harm to the person who dies, then the (conclusion of) deprivation theory is problematic.

(3) The Existence Requirement must be accepted, unless the proponents of the deprivation theory can offer at least one counterexample to defeat it.

(4) None of the examples the deprivation theorists offer decisively defeat the Existence Requirement.

(5) Therefore, the deprivation theory is problematic.

However, I suggest that this argument does not successfully refute the deprivation theory. The reason is as follows. Certainly, it would be ideal for the proponents of the deprivation theory to raise an counterexample to decisively defeat the Existence Requirement. If so, the Existence Requirement would be rejected directly. In a sense, I would say, death is just the best example. However, the fact that *none of the proponent's examples decisively defeats the Existence Requirement* does not mean that the Existence Requirement must be accepted. Without giving any reason for accepting the Existence Requirement, those opponents of the deprivation theory are simply begging the question. Indeed, in Chapter One, Section Two, I have shown that the Existence Requirement is problematic. If the Existence Requirement is rejected, then the claim that none of the proponent's examples decisively defeats the Existence Requirement should not be treated as a refutation of the deprivation theory.[13]

Another major challenge for the deprivation theory comes from the Lucretian symmetry argument. The challenge goes like this:

> Death is supposed to be an experiential blank that is bad insofar as it deprives the person who dies of the goods of life. Presumably, if one dies later rather than earlier, one can have more of the goods of life. But prenatal nonexistence seems in these ways precisely symmetric to death (conceived as posthumous nonexistence). That is, prenatal nonexistence is an indefinitely long experiential blank that is a deprivation of the goods of life: if one is born earlier rather than later, one can have more of the goods of life...But we do not regard prenatal nonexistence as a bad, misfortune, or harm; we do not tend to think it rational to regret it. Given this and the apparent symmetry between prenatal nonexistence and death (on the deprivation theory), it seems that we cannot consistently hold that death can be a bad thing for the person who dies, on the deprivation theory.[14]

At the first glance, it seems that the deprivation theory has been challenged if not refuted by the Lucretian symmetry argument. However, I argue to the contrary. The reason is that the Lucretian symmetry argument is incorrect (in Chapter Five, Section Two, I will discuss this argument in detail, and show why it is incorrect). If the Lucretian symmetry argument is fallacious, then the deprivation theory is not really refuted by this argument. However, this does not vindicate the deprivation theory. It means only that to question, or even to refute, the deprivation theory, we must seek other ways.[15]

3.2 A CRITIQUE OF THE DEPRIVATION THEORY

The outline of the deprivation theory in the last section is very general and basic. I therefore label it the 'primary deprivation theory'. There is still room for us to illuminate it in more detail, and to explore and criticise it further.

In his much-discussed paper "Death", Nagel, in order to support the claim that death is *always* an evil[16], adopts the following view (call it the 'logical' or 'imaginable' view). Nagel writes:

> Given an identifiable individual, *countless* possibilities for his continued existence are *imaginable*, and we can clearly conceive of what it would be for him to go on existing *indefinitely*...
>
> [A man's] existence defines for him an essentially *open-ended* possible future...Having been gratuitously introduced to the world by a collection of natural, historical, and social accidents, he finds himself the subject of a life, with an *indeterminate* and *not essentially limited* future. Viewed in this way, death, no matter how inevitable, is an abrupt cancellation of *indefinitely* extensive possible goods...If there is *no limit* to the amount of life that it would be good to have, then it may be that a bad end is in store for us all.[17] (My emphasis.)

This view is problematic. McMahan, for example, offers the following reason to reject it:

> If...the goods that would be possible for us were it not for death are conceived of as potentially *unlimited*, then it may seem that there is

nothing to prevent the conclusion that our losses in death are *infinite*. But then, if the loss involved in death is *infinite*, and if the badness of death consists in what it deprives us of, how can we explain the common and compelling belief that it is in general worse to die earlier rather than later—for example, that it is worse, or more tragic, when someone dies at thirty than it is when someone dies at eighty?[18] (My emphasis.)

To support McMahan, I offer another reason:

> Given the imaginable view, our losses in death are *infinite*. But then, if the loss involved in death is *infinite*, and if the badness of death consists in what it deprives us of, how can we explain the common and compelling belief that, in some circumstances, death is *not* a bad thing, or even a *good* thing, for the person who dies? For example, if a person P is suffering in excruciating agony from the final stage of cancer, we might rationally regard his death as a good thing for him. However, according to the imaginable view, even if P dies in this case, his death would be, all things considered, a grave harm or even a tragedy for him which sounds odd.

Put simply, the essential line of reasoning (or main point) of the imaginable view is: Death is *always* a harm or bad for the person who dies relative to the possibilities for good that one could imagine his life containing had that life continued.[19]

Here, McMahan gives the following two further reasons to reject this line of reasoning, and, thus, the imaginable view:

> (1) Simply to point out that there is an *imaginable* possible future life that a person might have had if he had not died seems insufficient to show that he met with a bad end. For we can also *imagine* possible future lives that the person might have had which would not have been worth living, relative to which his death could be judged not to be bad, or even to be good. Since desirable future lives and undesirable future lives are all equally *imaginable*, there seems to be no more reason to judge the person's death to be bad than there is to judge it to be good.
>
> (2) Unless there is some nonarbitrary way of selecting, from among the many *imaginable* lives the person might have had, the one

which can be considered the relevant alternative to death, then Nagel's focus on what would have been *imaginable* in the absence of death provides no basis for the evaluation of an individual's death.[20]

Accordingly, I think that the imaginable view should not be accepted. In other words, we should give up this *imaginable* line of reasoning involved in the imaginable view, when evaluating the badness of a person's death. In contrast, when evaluating the badness of a person's death, there seems to be a more acceptable line of reasoning—the 'factual (or practical)' line of reasoning. This line of reasoning is as follows:

> The possibilities for good of which a person is deprived by death are limited by the fact that, had he not died when and how he did, he would have been condemned by his biology and circumstances to die within a certain limited period of time thereafter.[21]

According to the above analyses, it is problematic for Nagel to claim that death is *always* a harm to the person who dies. Conversely, I think that it would be more proper to say that death is *generally* a harm to the person who dies.[22] In other words, a more reasonable conclusion of the deprivation theory is not: Death is *always* a harm to the person who dies. Rather, it is more appropriate to modify the conclusion to: Death is *generally* a harm to the person who dies.

Unfortunately, even if the primary deprivation theory is explicated or understood in this way, there are still some perplexing questions which need to be disentangled.

In his paper "Death and the Value of Life", McMahan claims that there is a difficult problem with the deprivation theory. He calls this problem the 'problem of specifying the antecedent'. I will discuss this alleged problem now.

The problem of specifying the antecedent is briefly expressed by McMahan as follows:

> Consider the case of a thirty-year-old man who died today of cancer. Call him Mort...[Given the deprivation theory], our evaluation of Mort's death must be based on a counterfactual conditional claim to the effect that 'such-and-such would have happened if...' The natural candidate for the antecedent of the counterfactual is, of

course, 'if he had not died'. But this is in fact hopelessly vague, for there are countless ways in which he might not have died.[23]

This 'problem' can be illustrated more concretely and fully as follows.

Take Mort's case as example. To evaluate his death, according to the deprivation theory, we must imagine that his death did not occur. To imagine that his death did not occur, we must imagine one of the following: (1) its cause did not occur, or (2) its cause did not lead to its expected effect.[24] Now, the alleged trouble here is that there are not only various ways of understanding what the cause of his death was, but there are also, for each way of conceiving of the cause of his death, various ways in which it would have been possible for the cause not to have operated.[25]

Suppose we specify cancer as the cause of Mort's death. Then in imagining that he might not have died, we can at least imagine:

(1) that he might never have been stricken with cancer in the first place;
(2) that he might have been cured of cancer; or
(3) that he might have lived on with cancer in a nonfatal form.[26]

Now, which one should we take? (1), (2), or (3)?

Further, the cause of Mort's death can also be understood as 'the immediate mechanism by which his death was brought about'—a haemorrhage or something else. And this will bring about a more serious trouble. To explain this, let us re-examine Mort's case.

If the cause of Mort's death is specified as cancer, and if the antecedent (i.e. 'if he had not died') is understood as 'had he been cured of cancer', then it is true that Mort's death can be regarded as a terrible tragedy for him. The reason is this. If Mort had not died when and how he did, he would have lived a long life. However, if the cause is identified as a haemorrhage, then his death was not tragic, or even perhaps was, *on balance*, a good thing for him. The reason is this. If he had not died when and how he did, he would have lived on for only a short period of time until his death would have certainly been brought about by some alternative mechanism associated with cancer. The brief future he would otherwise have had would have been excruciating for him.[27]

For further discussion, I offer another relevant case:

> John is twenty-five years old. He was run over by a car yesterday.
> Before he died at the hospital he had been suffering in extreme pain
> for 12 hours.

Similarly, in regard to John's case, we can make the following inference. If
the cause of his death is specified as the car accident, then it is true that
John's death can be regarded as a terrible tragedy for him. However, if the
cause is identified as, say, again, a haemorrhage, then his death was not
tragic, or even was, *on balance*, a good thing for him.

Anyway, *our choice of interpretation about the cause of a person's death
will make a difference to what our evaluation will be.*[28] Accordingly, a
person's death (e.g. Mort's death) would be, in a sense, a harm and not a
harm for him. This appears paradoxical.

To sum up, McMahan argues that, by conforming with the 'customary
method of specifying the antecedent', the deprivation theory would certainly
lead to the above paradoxical problem. To deal with this paradoxical
problem, he therefore suggests another method of specifying the antecedent
'*if he had not died*'. He believes that, by using his method of specifying the
antecedent, we can pick out the single, general, context-independent way of
evaluating a person's death. In other words, he believes that his method of
specifying the antecedent can tell us whether, all things considered, Mort's
(or John's) death was good or bad, and, therefore, this paradoxical problem
(i.e. the problem of specifying the antecedent) will be resolved.

Let me now briefly introduce McMahan's 'method of specifying the
antecedent'.

Firstly, McMahan defines the *transitive cause* of an event E as follows:

> If C is the immediate or proximate cause of E, then the transitive
> cause of E is the set of all the events that form part of the chain of
> causes leading to C.[29]

He continues to explain:

> This set is understood to be both complete and closed, in the sense
> that all and only the members of the set satisfy the following
> condition: if C_i is a member of the set and C_j is a cause of C_i, then
> C_j is a member of the set.[30]

On the basis of this definition, McMahan then states his method of specifying the antecedent:

> Let t be the time at which some person died. Our…evaluation of how bad or good his death was for him will be based on a counterfactual claim about what would have happened to him if he had not died at t. Let the antecedent of the relevant counterfactual be 'if the entire *transitive cause* of his death had not occurred…'[31] (My emphasis.)

At this point, I would like to demonstrate the shortcomings of McMahan's method of specifying the antecedent relative to Mort's case.

Firstly, suppose we single out the cause of Mort's death as a haemorrhage. According to McMahan's method of specifying the antecedent, to suppose that he might not have died is to suppose that the *transitive cause* of his haemorrhage did not occur. If we imagine that the *transitive cause* of his haemorrhage did not occur, then we must presumably imagine that he had not been stricken with cancer. Therefore, according to McMahan's method of specifying the antecedent, if Mort had not died from a haemorrhage, he would have lived a long life. That is, death in this case would be a harm or even a tragedy for him. Similarly, if we identify the cause of Mort's death as something else such as the degeneration of his liver functions, according to McMahan's method of specifying the antecedent, the evaluation of his death would be the same—a harm or even a tragedy for him. This can be shown as follows:

(1) If the *transitive cause* of the degeneration of his liver functions did not occur, then he would not have been stricken with cancer.
(2) If he had not been stricken with cancer, then he would have lived a long life.
(3) Therefore, if the *transitive cause* of the degeneration of his liver functions did not occur, then he would have lived a long life.
(4) Therefore, if he would otherwise have lived a long life, then his death would be a harm or even a tragedy for him.

In short, given McMahan's method of specifying the antecedent, the following conclusion would certainly be reached: Before a person had reached his biological life expectancy (100 years old or so), no matter how you single out the cause of his death (e.g. a haemorrhage or cancer or something else in Mort's case), his death would be *always* a harm or even a tragedy for him.

However, in certain circumstances, most of us (including most philosophers) believe that death can be a welcome release for the person who dies.[32] For example, when seeing Mort suffering from his terminal stage of cancer, we are inclined to think that living for him now means only torment. This is a very *general* evaluation of his condition. However, in taking McMahan's method of specifying the antecedent, we must say: 'Mort's death is a harm, or might even be a tragedy for him'. This conflicts *greatly* with our intuition.

Secondly, suppose we specify the cause of Mort's death as a haemorrhage. According to McMahan's method of specifying the antecedent, to suppose that he might not have died can be *merely* to suppose, in effect, that he had not been stricken with cancer.[33] However, there is no reason to prevent us from supposing that, (1) he had been cured of cancer, or (2) he had lived on with it in a nonfatal form. Certainly, it is natural for us also to suppose that, had he not have died, his death would have been brought about by some alternative mechanism associated with cancer. It seems to me that McMahan's method of specifying the antecedent is too narrow and limited to resolve the problem.

Let us now turn to what I shall call the 'customary method of specifying the antecedent'.

It is true, as McMahan points out, that, in conforming with the customary method of specifying the antecedent, our choice of interpretation of the *cause* of a person's death can make a dramatic difference in our evaluation of his death.[34] In other words, a person's death can be evaluated very differently depending on how we understand the circumstances of his not dying. In general, if we single out the cause of a person's death as causally closer to his death (i.e. to take a relatively narrower view of the cause of his death), then his death would not be a harm or even be a good thing for him.[35] Conversely, if we single out the cause of a person's death as causally further from his death (i.e. to take a relatively wider view of the cause of his death), then his death would be a harm or might even be a tragedy for him. These alternatives discomfort McMahan.

I think nevertheless that each of these perspectives of evaluation is very understandable and plausible. After all, it is reasonable to evaluate one event (or state of affairs) differently when considering it from *different* points of view. In some circumstances, we are inclined to take a relatively narrower view of the cause of a person's death; whereas in other circumstances, we are inclined to take a relatively wider view of the cause of that person's death.

When John's good friends hear about his bad news, most of them are inclined to feel that his death was a terrible tragedy for him—a relatively wider view. However, John's doctor friend, who had been seeing John suffering in agony during his final 12 hours and who also knew that further medical treatment could only extend John's suffering, might feel that death is a good thing for him—a relatively narrower view.[36]

On the other hand, when Mort's good friends, who had been seeing him suffering in excruciating agony from the final stage of cancer, are told that Mort has died, most of them would be inclined to feel that death was a welcome release for Mort—a relatively narrower view. However, in some circumstances, Mort's death can also be viewed as miserable. Suppose, for instance, that Mort's remote friend was merely told on the phone: 'Hi! Mort just died from the cancer two days ago!' Without any further information about Mort's death, this friend might only feel very sorry for him. He might think that if Mort had not died from the cancer, he would have been an excellent artist. That is to say, he might feel that death is a harm to Mort—a relatively wider view.

All of these supposed reactions sound *natural* and *reasonable*. In other words, the above evaluations of John's and Mort's deaths are not, as McMahan claims, paradoxical.

In order to further support his method of specifying the antecedent, McMahan offers another case:

> ...a young officer in the cavalry...was killed in the charge of the Light Brigade. This officer was among the leaders of the charge and was shot quite early by a soldier named Ivan. Suppose that, had he not been shot by Ivan, he would have been killed within a few seconds by a bullet fired by Boris, who also had him within his sights.[37]

As regards this case, McMahan, by following the customary method of specifying the antecedent, infers as follows:

> In the case of the cavalry officer...what we believe about what would have happened had he not died when and how he did depends on how we specify the cause of his death. If we single out the shot fired by Ivan as the cause and then ask what would have happened

had the cause not operated (e.g., because Ivan's hand shook, or his gun jammed), we get the answer that the officer would soon have been killed by Boris. We might, however, identify the cause of the officer's death differently—for example, as his being shot in the charge. If we ask what would have happened had he not been shot in the charge, the answer may well be that he would subsequently have led a long and happy life.[38]

He continues to analyse:

(1) If we specify the shot fired by Ivan as the cause of the officer's death, and if we *do* take the view of the customary method of specifying the antecedent, then we will certainly conclude that in this case all the officer lost in being shot by Ivan was *merely* a few seconds of life.
(2) Given the conclusion here, we must presumably accept the claim that the officer's actual death in this case was *hardly* a misfortune.[39]

The claim in (2) is a very bitter pill for McMahan to swallow. He, in fact, feels that the officer's death from the shot fired by Ivan should be regarded as a *grave* misfortune, depriving him of many years of life.[40] It is assumed that this feeling partly motivates him to offer his method of specifying the antecedent. Indeed, McMahan's method of specifying the antecedent can lead to the conclusion that the officer's death is a *grave* misfortune, depriving him of many years of life. This can be shown as follows:

(1) If we specify the cause of the officer's death as the shot fired by Ivan, then, according to McMahan's method of specifying the antecedent, to suppose that he might not have died is, thus, to suppose that the *transitive cause* of the officer's being shot by Ivan did not occur.
(2) If we imagine that the *transitive cause* of the officer's being shot by Ivan did not occur, then we must presumably imagine that the Crimean War (or at least the charge of the Light Brigade) did not occur.
(3) If the Crimean War did not occur, then the threat from Boris would not have occurred either.

(4) If the threat from Boris would not have occurred, then the officer would presumably have gone on to lead a long life.

(5) Therefore, his death from the shot fired by Ivan is a *grave* misfortune, depriving him of many years of life.

Again, I would like to address McMahan's method of specifying the antecedent and the customary method of specifying the antecedent relative to the cavalry officer's case.

It is extremely *natural* for us to specify the cause of the officer's death as 'the shot fired by Ivan'. In a sense, to single out the cause of the officer's death as 'the shot fired by Ivan' is more precise than to single it out as 'the charge of the Light Brigade (or his being shot in the charge)'. After all, it is the shot from Ivan that directly led to the officer's death. In addition, it can be imagined that the officer was not even wounded while attending this bloody charge.

By specifying the cause of the officer's death as the shot fired by Ivan, it would be very *natural* and *reasonable* to suppose that, had he not been shot by Ivan, he would have been killed within a few seconds by a bullet fired from someone else among Ivan's fellow soldiers such as Boris. Given this supposition, there is no doubt for the claim that all the officer lost in being shot by Ivan was *merely* a few seconds of life. Or put it more precisely, Ivan deprived the officer of merely a few *more* seconds of life. So far so good. Given that this claim is acceptable, it can therefore be concluded that the officer's *actual* death (from Ivan's shooting) was hardly a misfortune for him at all *in one sense*.

I believe that there is no problem with this inference, and, thus, I accept this conclusion.

McMahan might challenge my inference, and, therefore, the customary method of specifying the antecedent as follows:

> Well, after all, we may strongly feel that in this case the officer's death was a *grave* misfortune for him. But now, the conclusion which you have reached from the customary method of specifying the antecedent conflicts with this conviction. This is the reason why I want a different method of specifying the antecedent.

My response to this challenge is:

I agree that the officer's death was a grave misfortune for him *in one sense*. I also feel that way when thinking of his death from a certain point of view. But note that when I claim: 'The officer's *actual* death (from Ivan's shooting) in this case was hardly a misfortune for him at all *in one sense*', I do not rule out the possibility that the officer's death in this case was really a grave misfortune for him *in another sense*. Given the officer's death in this case could also be really a grave misfortune for him *in another sense* (I will show this later), there is no ground for you to reject the customary method of specifying the antecedent. On the other hand, when singling out the cause of the officer's death as the shot fired by Ivan which is quite natural, we are also inclined to feel, and have reason to believe, that Ivan deprived the officer of merely a few *more* seconds of life. After all, this is a fact. Thus, at least *in one sense*, it is true that the officer's death (from Ivan's shooting) in this case was hardly a misfortune for him. However, your method of specifying the antecedent completely ignores this *reasonable* and *natural* feeling.

According to the above analyses, it is definitely not true, as McMahan concludes, that the result brought about from the customary method of specifying the antecedent is a serious problem. Thus, the deprivation theorists should not, as McMahan suggests, give up this *natural* and *reasonable* customary method of specifying the antecedent. Conversely, given its shortcomings, I would suggest that McMahan's method of specifying the antecedent should be rejected.

If we accept the customary method of specifying the antecedent, then we must concede that, in some circumstances, not only can death be a very *small* harm to the person who dies (as shown in the cavalry officer's case), but also can death even be a *good* thing for the person who dies (as shown in Mort's case). Yet, according to the above analysis, in general, if we take a relatively narrower view of a person's death, then his death would not be a harm or might even be a good thing for him.

However, for the most part, we are inclined to take a relatively wider view of the cause of a person's death when evaluating his death. For example, *in general*, we do not specify the cause of John's death as a closer one such as a haemorrhage. On the contrary, we *generally* single out the cause of his death as the car accident. Therefore, our evaluation of a person's death would *generally* be that death is a harm to him.[41]

Accordingly, the conclusion of the deprivation theory should not be: Death is *always* a harm to the person who dies. Nor should it be: Death is *generally* a harm to the person who dies. Rather, it would be more accurate for the deprivation theory to conclude: Death is *generally* a harm to the person who dies *from a relatively wider view of the cause of his death* (or death *can* be a harm to the person who dies).[42]

Some people might be unsatisfied with this modified conclusion of the deprivation theory. They might view a person's death in his prime as *unconditionally* bad for him.[43] Indeed, there is good reason to feel that way. That is, it is true that a person's death in his prime is *always* unconditionally bad for him *in some sense*. To expose what this sense is, let us discuss McMahan's other case:

> Consider the following case. Joe is twenty-nine and a half years old. Schmoe has just turned thirty. Both are run over by a bus as they step off the curb. Our initial reaction is to think of both deaths as terribly tragic, Joe's being perhaps slightly more tragic than Schmoe's because of his slightly younger age. But suppose that, while Schmoe was in robust good health, it is discovered during the autopsy that Joe had a silent, symptomless, but invariably fatal disease that would have killed him within [six] months had he not been mown down by the bus. Our response to the discovery of this fact is to revise our initial assessment of the badness of Joe's death. Joe's death now seems considerably less bad than it would have been had he not had the condition since, given the fact that he had the condition, all he lost in being hit by the bus was at most [six] months of further life. Our revised response is thus to think that Schmoe's death was the more tragic of the two, other things being equal, even though he was older than Joe.[44]

When examining this case very carefully, we might find that there is a very puzzling problem with the deprivation theory. Let me illustrate this problem.

On the one hand, it is true, as McMahan asserts, that in this case Schmoe's death was the more tragic of the two. For in this case, what Schmoe lost in being hit by the bus was *much* more than what Joe lost in being hit by the bus.[45]

On the other hand, after thinking over this case, we might change our minds and believe that Joe's death was the more tragic of the two. This belief can be supported by the following argument:

(1) Suppose, as McMahan does in this case, that Joe and Schmoe had similar social circumstances and similar importance to other people, etc.

(2) Suppose also that Joe had not been killed in the bus accident for some reason such as someone's snatching him out of the path of the bus just at that very moment. He subsequently would continue to live for another six months until he died from his fatal disease *at the age of 30*. However, Schmoe, unfortunately, did die from the bus accident. He also died *at the age of 30*.

(3) Given (1), according to the deprivation theory, Joe's death from the fatal disease and Schmoe's death in the bus accident were equally tragic.

(4) In a sense, the bus accident had, in effect, brought forward Joe's death by six months.

(5) Since the earlier the death occurs, the more tragic it is (within a certain range), Joe's death in the bus accident was more tragic than his supposed death from the fatal disease.

(6) Given (3) and (5), Joe's death in the bus accident was more tragic than Schmoe's death in the bus accident.

(7) Therefore, in this case Joe's death was the more tragic of the two.

It appears that both views are confirmed by the deprivation theory. Now, the question here is, 'Whose death in the bus accident was the more tragic of the two? Joe's or Schmoe's?' It seems that we are now on the horns of a dilemma.

On the one hand, if we take the view that Schmoe's death in the bus accident was more tragic than Joe's death in the bus accident, then it seems that we also implicitly take the following view which is incorrect: The later the death comes, the more tragic it is. This can be shown as follows:

(i) Suppose that Schmoe's death in the bus accident was more tragic than Joe's death in the bus accident.

(ii) *'Schmoe's actual death in the bus accident'* and *'Joe's supposed death from his fatal disease'* were equally tragic (as shown above).

(iii) Given (ii), the supposition that *'Schmoe's actual death in the bus accident'* was more tragic than 'Joe's actual death in the bus accident' would entail that *'Joe's supposed death from his fatal disease'* was more tragic than 'Joe's actual death in the bus accident'.

(iv) Joe's supposed death from his fatal disease was later than his actual death in the bus accident (by six months).

(v) Therefore, the later the death comes, the more tragic it is.

On the other hand, if we take the view that Joe's death in the bus accident was more tragic than Schmoe's death in the bus accident, then it seems that we also implicitly adopt the following view which is also implausible: The less death deprives a person of, the more tragic it is. This can be shown as follows:

(i) Suppose that Joe's death in the bus accident was more tragic than Schmoe's death in the bus accident.

(ii) All Joe lost in being hit by the bus was six months of life; whereas Schmoe lost many years of life in being hit by the bus.

(iii) If (ii), then what death deprived Joe of in the bus accident was much *less* than what death deprived Schmoe of in the bus accident.

(iv) Now, Joe's death in the bus accident was more tragic than Schmoe's death in the bus accident, as supposed in (i).

(v) Therefore, the *less* death deprives a person of, the more tragic it is.

Again, whose death in a bus accident was the more tragic of the two?

To sort out this problem, I think we need to distinguish two notions which are usually conflated. Let me explain.

When considering the case of a person who dies prematurely, we can, and usually *do*, take two very different perspectives. Suppose someone P died in a car accident at the age of 30. In this case, the evaluation of the harm related to his death can be put as: His death *at the age of 30* is a harm to him. We are inclined to think that it is a terrible tragedy—a case of a young man prematurely cut down in his prime. On the other hand, the evaluation can also be put as: His death in the car accident is a harm to him. We are also inclined to think that the car accident (or this event) had, in fact, deprived him of many years of life. Indeed, we might think, had he not died in the car accident, he would have lived a long life.[46] Put simply, the evaluation of the harm related to P's death can be:

(1) P's death at the age of 30 (or the fact that P died at the age of 30) was a harm to him; or

(2) P's death event (or the event which brought about P's death) was a harm to him.

It is clear that the evaluation of *P's death event* (or the event which brought about P's death) here conforms entirely to the deprivation theory; whereas the evaluation of P's premature death (or the fact that P died prematurely) does not.

Indeed, the evaluation of P's premature death can be quite inconsistent with the evaluation of P's death event.[47] A person's premature death is *always* a harm to him (this will be discussed in Chapter Four, Section Two). However, a person's death event can be evaluated very differently depending on how we interpret this event (i.e. how we specify the cause of his death). According to the deprivation theory, the evaluation of a person's death event (or the event which brings about a person's death) can be: (1) a harm or even a tragedy for him, (2) a very *small* harm to him (i.e. hardly a misfortune for him), or even (3) a *good* thing for him.

On the other hand, these two notions—'the death event' and 'premature death'—are closely related. For one thing, in the case of a person who dies prematurely, his death event (or the event which brings about his death) will certainly bring about his premature death (or the fact that he dies prematurely). I think this can partly explain why these two notions are so easily conflated in an ambiguous formulation 'a person's death' by most recent philosophers.

To make the difference of these two notions more explicit and to reinforce the strong connection between them, let us re-examine Mort's and John's cases.

In Mort's case, if we interpret his death as caused by cancer, then his death event (or the event which brought about his death) was a harm to him. On the other hand, if we interpret the cause of his death as a haemorrhage (or the degeneration of liver functions), then his death event can be regarded as, *on balance*, a good thing for him. However, no matter how we interpret the cause of his death in this case (such as interpreting it as caused by cancer, a haemorrhage, or the degeneration of liver functions), these differently interpreted death events would certainly bring about the same result—his death *at the age of 30*. In other words, even though we interpret his death as caused by a haemorrhage (which was, on balance, a good thing for him), this interpreted death event would certainly bring about the fact that he died *at the age of 30*. And this fact was *always* a terrible tragedy for him. I think that perhaps this can explain why in some circumstances we *do* feel, and strongly believe, that a person's *death* (his death event or the event which brings about his death) is a welcome release for him; while we also feel that, after all, his *death* (his premature death or the fact that he dies prematurely) is a terrible tragedy for him.

In the cavalry officer's case, if we interpret his death as caused by the shot fired by Ivan, then his death event (or the event which brought about his death) was hardly a misfortune for him. This is because all he lost in this death event was merely a few seconds of life. However, although this interpreted death event was a very small harm to him, it would certainly lead to the fact that he died in his prime. And this fact was *always* a terrible tragedy for him. Therefore, it is possible that a person's premature death (or the fact that a person dies prematurely) is a terrible tragedy for him, although his 'death event' (on a certain interpretation) is a very small harm to him (i.e. hardly a misfortune for him).

By distinguishing 'a person's death event (or the event which brings about a person's death)' from 'a person's premature death (or the fact that a person dies prematurely)' I can now easily answer the question, 'Whose death in the bus accident was the more tragic of the two?'

My answer to the question is:

> Well, *in one sense* Joe's death is the more tragic of the two; *in another sense* Schmoe's death is the one which is the more tragic of the two. In any event, it very much depends on how we interpret the notion of *a person's death*. If the notion of a person's death is interpreted as *a person's premature death* (or the fact that a person dies prematurely), then Joe's death would be the more tragic of the two. The reason is simply that Joe was younger than Schmoe. On the other hand, if a person's death is interpreted as *a person's death event* (or the event which brings about a person's death), then Schmoe's death would be the one which is the more tragic of the two. The reason is this. What Schmoe lost in being hit by the bus is much more than what Joe lost in being hit by the bus.

As I mentioned above, the deprivation theory can be applied in evaluating a person's death event (or the event which brings about a person's death). Unfortunately, this theory has its limitations.

Firstly, as shown above, in the case of a person who dies prematurely, there is a very strong correlation between 'his death event (or the event which brings about his death)' and 'his premature death (or the fact that he dies prematurely)'—the former will certainly lead to the latter. However, the deprivation theory can apply only in evaluating the former. For instance, in Joe's case, in conforming to the deprivation theory, the conclusion we would reach is that Joe's death event (i.e. the bus accident) was not a terrible tragedy for him. It is impossible for the deprivation theory to reach the conclusion that Joe's premature death (or the fact that Joe died prematurely) was a terrible tragedy for him.

Secondly, if we claim that P can be harmed by his own death event (or the event which brings about his own death), then it is natural for us also to claim that he can be harmed by posthumous events. In fact, these two claims are so related that we are obliged either to affirm both or to deny both[48] (I will discuss posthumous harms in Chapter Four, Section Three). In short, there is a very strong correlation between 'the badness of the death event' and 'posthumous harms'. However, the deprivation theory cannot be extended to explain posthumous harms.

In brief, in the case of a person who dies prematurely, the following three notions are strongly connected: the badness of his premature death (or the fact that he dies prematurely), the badness of his death event (or the event which brings about his death), and his posthumous harms. Unfortunately, the deprivation theory can explain only the badness of his death event.

The limitations of the deprivation theory suggest that there might be scope for a comprehensive theory which can explain: (1) why a person's death event (or the event which brings about a person's death) is *generally* a harm to him from a relatively wider view of the cause of his death (or why a person's death event can be a harm to him), (2) why a person's premature death (or the fact that a person dies prematurely) is *always* a harm to him, and (3) why a person can be harmed *posthumously*. The deprivation theory might be a component of this comprehensive theory. In other words, the role of the deprivation theory, in this case, would be to offer a further interpretation of the reason this comprehensive theory gives for 'why a person's death event (or the event which brings about a person's death) is *generally* a harm to him from a relatively wider view of the cause of his death'. In Chapter Four, I will develop this comprehensive theory.

This theoretical limitation also suggests that it would be more precise to put the conclusion of the deprivation theory as: Death *as an event* is generally a harm to the person who dies from a relatively wider view of the cause of his death (or death *as an event* can be a harm to the person who dies).

CHAPTER FOUR

The Interest-Impairment Theory

In this chapter, I want to develop a comprehensive theory to account for: (1) the badness of the death event, (2) the badness of premature death, and (3) posthumous harms. For the purpose of this book, I will specifically address the justification of (1).

4.1 INTERESTS AND HARMS

The objective of this chapter is to explore a comprehensive theory which can explain: (1) why a person's death event (or the event which brings about a person's death) can be a *harm* to him, (2) why a person's premature death (or the fact that a person dies prematurely) is always a *harm* to him, and (3) why a person can be *harmed* posthumously. To reach this objective, first of all, I want in this section to give a brief, but reasonably precise, explication of the notion of *harm*. The reason for doing this is as follows.

In order to offer reasonable answers to these three questions, we should have a clear and appropriate understanding of what they mean. And a clear and appropriate understanding of what they mean is essentially based upon a reasonably precise explication of the notion of *harm*. Indeed, the explication of the notion of *harm* is a very important base or preparation for establishing any satisfactory answer to these three questions.

Before explicating the notion of harm, we need to explicate a more basic notion—*interest* on which the notion of harm relies.[1]

The notion of interest is ambiguous. It has at least two different meanings which can be expressed in the following two schemata:

(1) X is interested in Y.
(2) Y is in X's interests.[2]

To draw a conceptual distinction between these two, interest in the sense of (1) can be named as 'subjective interest (or psychological interest)', whereas interest in the sense of (2) as 'objective interest'. These two notions are clearly different. It is possible for someone to be interested in something that is not really in his *objective* interests. It is also possible for something to be in his *objective* interests regardless of the fact that he is not presently interested in it.

'Psychological interest' is not suitable to be used to explicate the sense of harm relevant here. For 'psychological interest' refers to an inclination to pay attention to something. In other words, the notion of psychological interest is too *subjective*. John Kleinig, for example, offers an example to show the difference between 'harm' and 'the thwarting of psychological interest'. He says:

> If, whenever I express a [psychological] interest in strawberries and cream, my wife harangues me on calories, cholesterol and coronaries, I may find myself losing [psychological] interest in strawberries and cream. But the 'invasion' of my [psychological] interest may have been all to the good [i.e. not a harm to me].[3]

To explicate the notion of harm, I suggest (following Kleinig) that we adopt '*objective* interest' which, following Feinberg, I explicate as follows:

> 'Objective interest' can be expressed as the form: 'Y is in X's interests'. 'Y is in X's interests' means 'X has a *justifiably claimed* stake in Y'. That is to say, Y is in X's interests when X has a *justifiably claimed* stake in Y. 'X has a stake in Y' is understood as 'X is likely to gain or lose from Y, because of some investment of energy or goods in Y or some project affected by Y, or because its outcome affects X advantageously or otherwise'.[4]

At first glance, there appears to be no conceptual difference or inconsistency between 'objective interest' and 'desire'. However, this is not true. We can in fact have an objective interest in something which is not an object of our desire. For example, having a stomach test is important for completely curing my stomach disease (i.e. it is in my objective interests), but it irks me very much (i.e. it is not an object of my desire). On the other hand, some objects of our desires are not in our objective interests. Indeed, we can even desire something which completely conflicts with our objective interests. For instance, drinking a dozen cans of Victoria Bitter beer with my good friends can be the object of my desire, but it would make me sick (i.e. it is not in my objective interests).[5]

In a sense, the notion of desire is more closely similar to the notion of *subjective* interest (psychological interest) than the notion of objective interest. Although 'desire' and 'psychological interest' have different intensions, they have almost the same extension. In addition, we are generally aware of both what we desire and what we are interested in. I think, this is partly because the notion of desire, like the notion of psychological interest, is also a *subjective* notion. Accordingly, 'desire' (with its *subjective* characteristics) is not suitable to be used to explicate harm either.

In terms of interest as characterised above, I would define harm as follows: *Harm is the impairment of objective interest.*[6]

Note that, in certain circumstances, our desires are really one of the important factors constituting our (objective) interests. Sometimes, a desire can even be the essential factor for constituting an (objective) interest. Besides, most of the time we desire what is in our (objective) interests. This really makes these two concepts tightly linked. Perhaps, this is part of the reason why the desire-thwarting theory is suggested. But note further that, even in these circumstances, it is not just the nonfulfilment of what we desire that accounts for the *harm*. I claim that it is the nonfulfilment of what we desire together with the fact what we desire is in our (objective) interests that accounts for *harm*.

To clarify the definition of harm I suggest here, I want to discuss another two different definitions of harm which are very similar to mine, but which are defective.

The first one is from Feinberg. Feinberg is quite right when he points out that 'harm' is better defined a more *objective* way. He says, '... harm to an interest is better defined in terms of the *objective* blocking of goals [desires]...than in subjective terms...'[7] (My emphasis.) He offers a definition which looks just like mine—harm is the violation of one of a person's interests.[8] However, he still confuses *interest* with *desire*. Or more precisely speaking, he explicates *interest* (and thus *harm*) by using *desire.*[9] This can be shown as follows.

Feinberg introduces a pair of conceptions:

(1) Want-fulfilment: the coming into existence of that which is desired.

(2) Want-satisfaction: the pleasant experience of contentment or gratification that normally occurs in the mind of the desirer when he believes that his desire has been fulfilled.[10]

Feinberg claims that interest (and thus, harm) should be defined by *want-fulfilment*, but *not want-satisfaction*. He says, '... an interest [and thus, harm] is...best defined in terms of the objective fulfilment of well-considered wants rather than in terms of subjective states of pleasure.'[11] (My emphasis.)

Although Feinberg is aware that 'harm' is better defined in a more *objective* way, unfortunately he does not make his definition *objective* enough. Interpreting interest in terms of *want-fulfilment*, in reality, Feinberg still uses *desire* (with the *subjective* characteristics) to define 'harm'. Since desire is *not* suitable to be used to explicate harm as argued above, Feinberg's definition of harm is seriously flawed.

The second different definition of harm is from Kleinig who defines harm as *the impairment of a (human) being's welfare interests.*[12] There are two main problems with this definition.

The first problem is as follows. By 'welfare interests' Kleinig means those interests which are indispensable to the pursuit and fulfilment of happiness or well-being. Welfare interests are seen, by Kleinig, as opportunities for happiness or well-being.[13] Because *well-being* varies between cultures that would make *welfare* a variable notion. This makes the notion of welfare interests difficult to apply.

The second more serious difficulty is this. According to Kleinig's definition of harm, harm is done only when welfare interests are impaired. Welfare interests are specified by Kleinig as 'bodily and mental health, normal intellectual development, adequate material security, stable and non-superficial inter-personal relationships, and a fair degree of liberty'.[14] Apparently, there can be no welfare interests (as mentioned above) left after we die. Given this, it is impossible for any events happening after our death to impair our welfare interests (so understood). Therefore, according to Kleinig's definition of harm, we cannot be harmed any more after we die. In short, Kleinig's definition of harm fails to accommodate posthumous harms.

To my criticism, Kleinig might reply, 'This is a *difficulty* only for those who believe in posthumous harms'. However, I will argue that there can be posthumous harms in this chapter, Section Three.

There are another two different kinds of harm which are the specialised adaptations of the harm I define above: (1) moral harm, and (2) legal harm. However, neither of them is consistent with our general understanding of harm.

Moral harm is understood as the impairment of one's *moral* interests. In terms of moral harm, only *acts* are harmful and only *people* do moral harm. Thus, according to the notion of moral harm, if a tree, weakened by termites, topples onto my leg, breaking it, the leg will be said to suffer damage or injury, but not harm.[15] I am hurt physically but because the tree is *not* an agent, I am not harmed. This is clearly inconsistent with our general understanding of harm. Kleinig also offers the following example to illustrate the unreasonableness of the notion of moral harm:

> If the neck of a two-year old child is broken, according to the general understanding of harm, he is unequivocally harmed. However, according to the notion of 'moral harm', the child is harmed, only if his morally good interests are impaired...[16]

On the other hand, according to the notion of legal harm, harm is understood as the violation of a *legally* protected interest. This interpretation of harm can lead to the following strange consequence: 'If X trespasses on Y's land, he has done Y harm insofar as he has violated Y's legally protected interest in the exclusive use and enjoyment of his land.'[17]

In short, the sense of harm which is crucial is distinct from these two kinds of harm.

Someone might challenge my definition of harm by raising the following two cases:

> Case One. A crime boss invests large amounts of money and energy in an attempted bank robbery, but his attempt is foiled. According to your definition, it seems that the crime boss is harmed.[18]

> Case Two. I buy a lottery ticket, but I do not win one million dollars. Had I won one million dollars, I would have benefited, but my failure to benefit shouldn't be regarded as harmful. However, it

seems that according to your definition, winning one million dollars is in my interests, so I am harmed.

In these two cases, I agree that neither the crime boss nor the lottery player is harmed. However, this does not mean that my position is rejected. To rebut this challenge, it is very important to distinguish *interest* from *benefit*. Feinberg, by using another case, draws a distinction between them:

> Thus, if I have an annual salary of one hundred thousand dollars [which I am entitled to have], and my employer gives me a fifty thousand dollar raise, I benefit substantially from his largesse. If he fails to give me a raise, I am not so benefited, but surely not harmed either...If he reduces me to five thousand [without any acceptable reason]...however, he not merely fails to benefit me, he causes me harm...[19]

I completely agree with Feinberg's judgement here. However, the reason he gives for reaching his conclusion is flawed. He writes:

> We harm a man when we deny or deprive him of something he needs; we fail to benefit him (merely) when we deny or deprive him of some good he does not need. An unneeded good is something a person wants which is not necessary for his welfare, something he can do without.[20]

According to this statement, harm is the thwarting of *need*. And *need* is interpreted as 'something which is necessary for his *welfare*'. Thus, here Feinberg, like Kleinig, also adopts the *welfare-impairment* definition of harm. Since this definition is problematic, as was argued above, Feinberg's reason for reaching his above conclusion is problematic as well. By following this problematic reason, we can even lead to the following ridiculous conclusion:

> Since my son's life is not necessary for my welfare, I am not harmed by his death in a car accident. However, according to Feinberg, if my boss reduces my salary to five thousand, then he not merely fails to benefit me, he causes me harm.

It is time now for me to theoretically illuminate these two concepts—
'benefit'and 'interest':

> 'Y is a *benefit* to me' means 'I have a stake in Y'; whereas 'Y is in
> my *interests*' means 'I have a *justifiably claimed* stake in Y'. Thus,
> *not* every benefit is in my interests. On the other hand, *every interest
> is a benefit.* 'Justifiably claimed' can be interpreted as meaning
> 'entitled'. Consequentially, 'interest' can be understood as 'entitled
> benefit'.

On the basis of this analysis, I can now reasonably respond to these three
cases.
      With regard to Case One, I will reply as follows:

> The crime boss is not entitled to benefit from the robbery money.
> Robbery is both illegal and immoral. That is, the robbery money is
> not in his (legitimate) interests, although it might be to his benefit.
> Therefore, he is not harmed from his failing to get the money.

Case Two is a little bit more difficult than Case One, because playing lotto is
neither illegal nor immoral. I can still reply as follows:

> Yes, playing lotto is neither illegal nor immoral. However, the one
> million dollars is still not in the lotto player's interests. It is not the
> case that the one million dollars should belong to him. Neither is it
> certain that he will win the one million dollars. For one thing, every
> lotto player is a potential beneficiary who may win one million
> dollars. If so, then it is acceptable for a lotto player not to win one
> million dollars. It is in this sense I claim that failing to win one
> million dollars is not in violation of his entitled benefits (i.e. it is not
> in violation of his interests). That is, although the one million dollars
> is to his benefit, it is not in his interests. Therefore, if he does not
> win it, he is not harmed.

By the same token, I can also explain Feinberg's case:

> A fifty thousand dollar raise is not in my interests, because it is not
> an entitled benefit. Thus, I am not harmed when my boss fails to give

me a raise. On the other hand, the salary is in my interests, because it is an entitled benefit. Thus, if he reduces me to five thousand, he not merely fails to benefit me, he causes me harm.

Accordingly, I completely agree with William Grey, who has pointed out to me that if I do not win lotto, then I am not harmed. However, once I win the money and the money is stolen, then I am harmed.

4.2 THE HARMS OF THE DEATH EVENT AND PREMATURE DEATH

In the last section, I have briefly and clearly explicated the pair of notions: *interest* and *harm*. Most importantly, according to this explication, I have also reached the conclusion: *Harm is the impairment of interest* (call this the 'interest-impairment principle'). On the basis of this principle, I want, in this section, to argue that: (1) a person's *death event* (or the event which brings about a person's death) can be a harm to him, and (2) a person's *premature death* (or the fact that a person dies prematurely) is *always* a harm to him. After this, in the next section, I want, on the basis of the interest-impairment principle, to continue to argue that a person can be harmed *posthumously*. These three arguments are the essential components of the comprehensive theory mentioned above. Since this theory is essentially based on the interest-impairment principle, I therefore call it the '*interest-impairment theory*'.

Let us explore this theory now.

Can the *death event* be a harm to the person who dies? Or can a person's *death event* (or the event which brings about a person's death) be a harm to him? To this question, my answer is, 'Yes, of course!' But why?

There are two main theories which try to offer a reason for an affirmative answer to this question: the desire-thwarting theory and the deprivation theory. According to the analysis in Chapter Two, Section One, an appropriate expression of the desire-thwarting theory is:

(1) Something is a harm or misfortune for us if it thwarts any of our desires.
(2) Death thwarts certain kind(s) of our *unconditional* desires.
(3) Therefore, death is a harm or misfortune for us.

I have rejected the desire-thwarting theory in Chapter Two, Section Two. Further, I argued, in the last section, that 'harm' could not be explained by 'desire'. However, in a very special sense, the desire-thwarting theory *does* explain some harms. The reason is as follows.

All healthy and rational men have some projects and plans for their future (i.e. future-oriented desires). Some of them are so-called (future-oriented) dependent *unconditional* desires. For example, someone P might desire to produce an excellent book or a beautiful art object before the year 2001 *by himself*, or wish to travel in Mongolia and cross a big desert by riding camels with his girlfriend by the year 2001 and so on. Apparently, all these (future-oriented) dependent *unconditional* desires will be completely thwarted at a stroke by his *death event* (or the event which brings about his death). Since harm, as we have already emphasised above is understood as the *impairment of interest* and we all have an interest in not being thwarted in our desires, it follows that the thwarting of our desires is one species of harm. Accordingly, in this very sense, the *death event* is a harm to us, since the *death event* is the thwarting of all our (future-oriented) dependent *unconditional* desires. Therefore, in this sense, P's *death event* (or the event which brings about P's death) is a harm to him.

But note that a harm caused by a death event in this sense is only a *second order* or *indirect* one. Basically, it is a harm of a relatively trivial or unimportant kind. To really justify the claim that P's death event (or the event which brings about P's death) can be a harm to him, a *direct* and *positive* reason is needed. This direct and positive reason is given by the 'interest-impairment theory *of the harm of the death event*' which I will now discuss.

First of all, it is claimed that, in general, the continuation of our lives *in the way we normally lived (before)* is in our interests.[21] The reason for this claim is:

(1) Life (or being alive) is a precondition of a variety of happiness (goods) and miseries (bads).

(2) If our lives continue (in the way we normally lived), then the goods we will have will *generally* outweigh the bads we will have. That is, if our lives continue (in the way we normally lived), then we will *generally* have a good life.

(3) Given (2), the continuation of our lives (in the way we normally lived) is *generally* in our interests.

Since the claim that the continuation of our lives *in the way we normally lived* is generally in our interests is the starting point of the interest-impairment theory *of the harm of the death event*, it is very important to further illuminate and justify it. Let us do this by examining the three points discussed above which constitute the reason for this claim.

The requirements for (1) to be the case are clear. Feinberg, for example, offers the following reason to support the claim that life (or being alive) is a precondition of a variety of happiness (goods). He writes:

> ...unless we continue [being] alive, we have no chance whatever of achieving those goals that are the ground of our ultimate interest...[Being alive] is...an indispensable condition for the advancement of most, if not all, of the ulterior interests that constitute our good.[22]

Of course, life (or being alive) is also a precondition of a variety of miseries (bads). In short, as Sumner says, 'Life is the condition of all goods, but alas it is also the condition of all evils'.[23]

Let us now move on to (2) and (3). A simple and clear reason for (2), and thus (3), can be put as follows.

Apparently, with the continuation of our lives (in the way we normally lived), in general, we will have a good life. After all, life is *generally* good as assumed in Introduction. Given this, the continuation of our lives (in the way we normally lived) is *generally* in our interests.

For a further understanding of this reason, let me specify it in more detail as follows.

It is easy for us to reasonably imagine, according to P's current condition, some possible goods (happiness) in his continuing life. For example, he will keep enjoying a happy family life; have more exciting trips; or even write some good philosophical books and so on. Of course, we can also reasonably imagine, according to P's current condition, some possible bads or even afflictions in his continuing life. For instance, he will keep suffering the problem with his stomachache; suffer more and more work pressure; or even gradually have a worsening relationship with his son and so on. Upon the whole, we would think that in P's continuing life (in the way he normally lived), the possible future goods will *generally* outweigh the possible future bads. Therefore, it is believed that P's continuing life (in the way he normally lived) will *generally* be good for him. Given this, the continuation of his life (in the way he normally lived) will be *generally* in his interests.[24]

Given that the continuation of P's life (in the way he normally lived) is *generally* in his interests and given that *harm is the impairment of interest*, we can therefore reach the conclusion: P's death event (or the event which brings about P's death) from a relatively wider view of the cause of his death is *generally* a harm to him. This conclusion can be derived as follows:

(i) Suppose P died at time T. It is certain that P's *death event* (or the event which brought about P's death) from a relatively wider view of the cause of his death directly blocked the continuation of his life (in the way he normally lived).

(ii) *Generally*, the continuation of P's life (in the way he normally lived) was in his interests (as shown above).

(iii) If the continuation of his life (in the way he normally lived) was *generally* in his interests, then P's death event (or the event which brought about P's death) from a relatively wider view of the cause of his death, which blocked the continuation of his life (in the way he normally lived), would *generally* have impaired P's interest.

(iv) *Harm is the impairment of interest.*

(v) Therefore, P's death event (or the event which brought about P's death) from a relatively wider view of the cause of his death, was *generally* a harm to him. Or at least, P's death event (or the event which brought about P's death) could be a harm to him.[25]

Call this argument the 'interest-impairment theory *of the harm of the death event*'.

In fact, the above analysis concerning the badness of P's death event (or the event which brought about P's death) from a relatively wider view of the cause of his death has implicitly included an assumption which can be briefly explicated as follows:

(i) The badness of P's death event (from a relatively wider view of the cause of his death) essentially consists in its bringing about the curtailment of P's life which is a harm or might even be a tragedy for P. That is, it essentially consists in its impairing P's interest in the continuation of his life.

(ii) The badness of the curtailment of P's life essentially consists in its depriving P of possible future goods.

Basically, from (i), we can detect the interest-impairment principle, while (ii) is actually the re-emergence of the deprivation theory in an extended form. Indeed, the interest-impairment theory *of the harm of the death event* is the fusion of the interest-impairment principle and the deprivation theory. In other words, it is the extension of the deprivation theory by including the interest-impairment principle.

It should be emphasised here that the continuation of our lives may *not* always be in our interests. In certain circumstances, the continuation of our lives can be miserable (i.e. not in our interests, *all things considered*).[26] Therefore, death as an event is *not* always, all things considered, a harm to us. For example, when one is suffering from a terminal, excruciatingly painful illness, the continuation of his life in this case can be rationally regarded as, all things considered, a harm or might even be a tragedy for him. Consequently, the death event, which ends the continuation of a life in this case, would be rationally regarded as a welcome release for him. In general, as I have shown in Chapter Three, Section Two, death as an event (from a relatively *narrower* view of the causes of death) would end the continuation of our lives in miserable circumstances. Therefore, death as an event (from a relatively *narrower* view of the cause of death) would, all things considered, generally *not* be a harm or even be a *good* thing for the person who dies.

Let us now move on to another question, 'Can a person's premature death (or the fact that a person dies prematurely) be a harm to him?' With regard to this question, my answer is, 'Yes, of course!' However, this affirmative answer is challenged by Gisela Striker.

Striker embraces a position which disregards or even rules out the importance of duration (i.e. the length of life) in considering or evaluating the badness (or harm) of premature death. She writes:

> ...*duration* is not really the issue. What we are rightly concerned about when we are afraid of dying [premature death] is *completeness* as opposed to incompleteness, and that is only incidentally a matter of sheer length of time.[27] (My emphasis.)

To illustrate her point, Striker offers an analogy by way of example:

> The eighteen year old who wants to continue living is like someone who has watched the first act of an opera and is justifiably annoyed if the performance breaks off at this point. He is angry, *not because he had thought he was going to spend three hours instead of only*

one [i.e. short duration], but because he wanted to see the entire opera, not just a part of it [i.e. incompleteness]...
    And if our lives are in some way comparable to operas, one might argue that...an opera does not necessarily get better from being longer. Similarly, then, our lives will not be better for being longer...[28] (My emphasis.)

My response to Striker is as follows. Suppose, following Striker's line of reasoning, that *completeness* is a vital factor in considering or evaluating whole life's happiness and well-being, and, thus, the badness (or harm) of premature death.[29] Nevertheless *duration* is also a very important factor in considering or evaluating the badness of premature death. The reason for this is as follows.

Firstly, it is apparent that the fulfilment of our (well-considered) life plans or projects is in our interests.[30] For these to be fulfilled (i.e. to live a *complete* life), we must have a sufficient life span. As Striker herself says, 'a very short life could not possibly be complete.'[31] In this sense, *duration* is still very important. Using Striker's analogy, in only one hour, the entire opera cannot be performed.

Secondly, if P dies prematurely, we will normally feel sorry for him. We might feel pity for him when, as Striker emphasises, we think of all his life plans and projects that have been broken off. We might also feel pity for him when we simply think of the fact that he cannot even live the normal lifespan of a human being (without any knowledge about his life plans and projects). To clarify this point, let me use Striker's example again. If the opera performance breaks off at the first act of the opera, one can be disappointed because one wanted to see the entire opera, not just a part of it. However, one can also be disappointed because one had planned to spend three hours there, instead of only one, particularly if the opera ticket cost $500.

Perhaps Striker would reply, 'To see the entire opera (i.e. *completeness*) is more important than to spend the whole three hours there (i.e. *duration*).' I agree with this. However, the latter is still important. In other words, *duration* is also a very important factor when we consider or evaluate the badness of premature death.

Let me now explore the reason (namely, the 'interest-impairment theory *of the harm of premature death*') why a person's premature death (or the fact that a person dies prematurely) is *always* a harm to him.

As human beings, it is *always* a benefit for us to live a normally healthy life until our natural biological life expectancy (or at least to live the normal lifespan of human beings in a normally healthy condition). And we, as human beings, are *entitled* to have this benefit. In other words, to live a normally healthy life until our natural biological life expectancy (or at least to live the normal lifespan of human beings in a normally healthy condition) is *always* in our interests.

Suppose P died in his prime. His premature death (or the fact that he died prematurely) would entail that he died before reaching his natural biological life expectancy, which it was *always* in his interests to do. Therefore, his premature death would have certainly impaired his interest in living a normally healthy life until reaching his natural biological life expectancy (or at least living the normal lifespan of human beings in a normally healthy condition). Given that *harm is the impairment of interest*, P therefore has been harmed by his premature death. According to this analysis, the following conclusion can be reached: The fact that a person dies before reaching his natural biological life expectancy is not merely a harm to him, but is *always* a harm to him.

Given this conclusion, it is still the case that the death of a young person, who is terminally ill with the prospect of only a few weeks of intense suffering, is a harm to him in the sense in which premature death is *always* a harm—even though, all things considered, his death (event) may be good for him.

A related issue is: Does the fact that we can live a life only until our natural biological life expectancy (say, 100 years old) constitute a harm or misfortune for us? Some philosophers believe that it is. McMahan, for example, has devised an ingenious defence of this position. He says:

> Consider, for example, the case of a person who dies from extreme old age, at the biological limits of human life [at 100 years old]. Call this person Gerry...Gerry suffers a serious misfortune. Indeed, it is compatible with the view that ultimately we *all* suffer a great misfortune—even those of us who live the longest, richest lives. This is not the best of all possible worlds. We are all subject to ageing beyond maturity, disease, injury, death, and so on. Were it not for these various evils, each of us would enjoy the prospect of an indefinitely extensive succession of possible goods...
>
> Even though those who gain more from life than most of us do suffer a misfortune when they die...[32]

The position McMahan takes—the fact that we *do* live a life only until our natural biological life expectancy (say, 100 years old) is a harm or misfortune for us—can be rejected, by using his own example, as follows.

I suggest that McMahan has confused two different notions—*benefit* and *interest*—which leads him to this mistaken conclusion. It would be appropriate, in this case, to say, 'It is to Gerry's benefit for him to live beyond 100 years'. However, to live beyond 100 years is definitely *not* in his interests. For, as a human being, he is not *entitled* to have that benefit. Therefore, his death at 100 is not a harm or misfortune (or at the very least is *hardly* a harm or misfortune) for him. To illustrate this point, let us look again at a modification of an example which Feinberg offers.

> Thus, if I have an annual salary [life] of one hundred thousand dollars [100 years], and my employer [God] gives me a fifty thousand dollar [50 year] raise, I benefit substantially from this largesse. If he [God] fails to give me a raise, I am not so benefited, but surely not harmed either...If he [God] reduces me to five thousand [50 years]...however, he [God] not merely fails to benefit me, he [God] causes me harm...[33]

In short, once we are living in this world, the fact that we live a life only until our natural biological life expectancy should not be seen as a harm or misfortune for us. At most, perhaps, it is a matter of regret for us.

According to the above discussion, it is claimed that the death of an elderly person who has led a full and worthwhile life is not a great misfortune for him.

Let me now review the results so far of my examination of the issues about death:

> (1) Death *as an event* (from a relatively *closer* view of the cause of death) is generally *not* a harm or may even be a good thing for the person who dies.
> (2) The fact that we can live a life only until our natural biological life expectancy is *not* a harm or misfortune for us.

Most importantly, I have reached the following conclusions:

> (1) A person's premature death (or the fact that a person dies prematurely) is *always* a harm to him.

(2) Death as an event (from a relatively wider view of the cause of death) is *generally* a harm to the person who dies. Or at least, *death (as an event) can be a harm to the person who dies.*

Let us move on to another very important question, 'Can a person be harmed posthumously?'

4.3 POSTHUMOUS HARMS AND THE MISSING SUBJECT PROBLEM

Can persons be harmed by posthumous events? That is, can an event that occurs after a person's death count as a harm or misfortune for him? With regard to this question, Ernest Partridge comments:

> Plausible, well-considered arguments can be presented to support either affirmative or negative answers to [this question]. And yet…either response to [this question] may appear, for clear and evident reasons, to be strange and outlandish; in a word, [this question seems] to be such that no answer can put us fully at ease…
>
> …the issue of 'posthumous interests' and 'posthumous harms' presents 'a hard case' for disputants on either side of the issue.[34]

Given this, before offering the answer to this question, I would invite you to consider the following three relevant cases.

> Case One. Bill Brown promises his dying father that he will bury him in the family plot when he dies. Bill instead sells his father's corpse to a medical school for dissection by students, since he needs money for gambling.[35]

> Case Two. A philosopher spends his entire life working on a metaphysical system that he believes to be, and desperately wants to be, the Truth about reality. And it is! Unfortunately, a disgruntled neighbor burns the philosopher's house down the day after his death, and his writings are destroyed. Even worse, he never revealed his metaphysical views to anyone; so his system is irretrievably lost, and

the philosopher is remembered only by a few friends and the hostile neighbor.[36]

Case Three. After John's death, an enemy cleverly forges documents to 'prove' very convincingly that John was a philanderer, an adulterer, and a plagiarist, and communicates this 'information' to the general public that includes his widow, children, and former colleagues whose good opinion he coveted and cherished.[37]

In the face of Case One, our intuition tells us that Mr. Brown has been badly harmed. As to Case Two, we are inclined to think that the neighbour's vicious action harms the philosopher (as well as philosophy!) Similarly, in Case Three, most people, I believe, are strongly inclined to feel that John has been harmed by such libels. Indeed, in considering these three cases, it is very difficult for us to conclude that it is impossible to be harmed by posthumous events. I, therefore, support the position that it *is* possible to be harmed posthumously. However, in order to affirm the validity of this position, it is necessary to explain what underlies these intuitions (i.e. to offer further theoretical support). Let me now explore this theoretical reason (namely, the 'interest-impairment theory *of posthumous harms*').

First of all, I take it that some of a person's interests can survive the death of the person and are still capable of being blocked.[38]

Persons can, in fact, have different kinds of interests. Some of these interests die with them. These are the kinds of interests which can no longer be promoted or harmed by posthumous events. These include most of their self-regarding (dependent) interests, those based, for example, on personal achievement and personal enjoyment.[39] However, there are still some other kinds of interests which can survive their owner's death, and can be promoted or defeated by events subsequent to that death. In other words, after a person dies, it is still possible for some of his interests to be promoted or dashed. For example, a person's reputation or the well-being of his children can still be promoted or harmed by events subsequent to his death. Indeed, a person's interest in his good reputation might be defeated by posthumous events as Case Three shows. Similarly, his interest in the well-being of his children could be defeated or harmed after his death by other parties overturning his will, or by thieves and swindlers who cheat his heirs of their inheritance.[40]

According to the above analysis, it seems that the claim that some of a person's interests can survive the death of the person and thus be harmed, is fairly plausible. However, this position is challenged by its opponents who point out the following difficulty:

> (1) All interests are the interest of some persons or other. In other words, there must be a subject for there to be any interest.
> (2) Death is the cessation of one's existence. After death, there is no longer a subject.
> (3) Therefore, there are no surviving interests.[41]

I think that this is a very simple and perhaps the most powerful argument against the possibility of posthumous harms. Indeed, we are obliged to admit both premise (1) and premise (2) in this argument. After all, it would be absurd to say there are interests (floating in the air) without any subject. It is also very difficult to accept the view that all interests are the interests of some Absolute Mind. To adopt this view would be, says Feinberg, 'a metaphysical assumption that is uneconomical.'[42] Besides, it is also true, in a sense, that after death there is no longer a subject.

Basically, this argument can be derived from the Epicurean argument. It *does* indeed pose a problem for the claim that a person's interests *can* survive the death of the person and thus, can be frustrated. Call this problem the 'missing subject problem concerning posthumous harms'. I believe that the solution of the missing subject problem concerning posthumous harms is an essential theoretical task for writers who have strong theoretical incentives for defending the position that a person's interests *can* survive the death of the person and therefore, are still capable of being frustrated. In other words, our task is to locate the subject of these surviving interests (and thus, the corresponding harms), given the premises (1) and (2).

Apparently, these surviving interests are not themselves the true subjects of these surviving interests and thus, the corresponding harms, because, as Feinberg points out, 'that suggests a bizarre reification, as if each interest were a little person in its own right.'[43] To locate where the true subject of these surviving interests, and thus the corresponding harms is, it is useful to examine George Pitcher's illustration of two ways of describing a dead person.

Pitcher points out that there are two different things a person might do if he sets out to describe a friend of his who is now dead:

> (i) He can describe the dead friend as he was at some stage of his life—i.e. as a living person.

(ii) He can describe the dead friend as he is now, in death—mouldering, perhaps, in a grave.[44]

Pitcher notes, 'in (i) we may say that there is a description of an *ante*-mortem person after his death, while in (ii) there is a description of a *post*-mortem person after his death.'[45]

Clearly, it would be utterly absurd to assert that the interests harmed by events that occur after the moment a person's nonexistence commences are interests of the decaying body he left behind. This contradicts premise (1) and should therefore be rejected. If so, then it is natural for us to think that the subject of the surviving interests and thus the corresponding harms, must be the *living* person who was formerly but no longer is with us—an *ante*-mortem person referred to after his death. With regard to this view, Pitcher comments as follows:

> I maintain that although both ante-mortem and post-mortem persons can be described after their death, only ante-mortem persons can be wronged [or harmed] after their death. Suppose, for example, that Mrs. Blue, now dead, *was* not in the least anti-Semitic, but that her spiteful neighbor now maliciously asserts that she *was*. This charge is a lie and since it is a lie about a person who is now dead, it may be said to constitute a wrong [or a harm] perpetrated against a dead person. Her neighbor wrongs [or harms] the dead Mrs. Blue when he falsely states that she *was* anti-Semitic. But he wrongs [or harms] the ante-mortem Mrs. Blue, not the post-mortem Mrs. Blue: he falsely charges that Mrs. Blue when alive *was* anti-Semitic, and so it is the living Mrs. Blue who *is* wronged [or harmed]. Her neighbor says nothing either true or false about Mrs. Blue as she is now, in death. Indeed, it would be nonsense to suggest that Mrs. Blue, after her death—the post-mortem Mrs. Blue—could be anti-Semitic.[46] (My emphasis.)

Feinberg says also:

> All antemortem persons are subject not only to being described, but also to being wronged after their deaths, by betrayals, broken promises, defamatory lies, and the like, but no 'posthumous person' can be wronged at all. (How could one break a promise to a corpse, or wrong the corpse by misdescribing it?) Posthumous persons

cannot be harmed either, for no 'mere thing' can be harmed directly in its own right, but only in a 'derivative sense'.[47]

To further support the claim that the subject of the surviving interests and thus, the corresponding harms must be the *living* person who no longer is with us—an *ante*-mortem person after his death—let us look back the above three cases. In Case One, when young Brown sells his father's corpse to the medical school, he breaks a promise he made to his father before the old man died: so it is the living Mr. Brown who *is* harmed by his son's action. In Case Two, it is the philosopher who actually worked on a metaphysical system establishing the Truth about reality—i.e. the living philosopher—who *is* harmed by his disgruntled neighbour's destroying all his writings. Similarly, in Case Three, it is the living John who *is* harmed by such libels. In short, it is impossible to harm a *post-mortem* person. Post-mortem persons are, if anything, just so much detritus; and detritus cannot be harmed.[48] Note that, in Case Three, John's interest in his good reputation was not thwarted by his death itself, but by events that occurred afterward.

Accordingly, it may now be concluded that the subject of the surviving interests and thus the corresponding harms, is the *ante-mortem* person. Since I have located the subject of the surviving interests and thus the subject of the corresponding harms, I may, therefore, claim that a person can be harmed by posthumous events.

In fact, as Raymond A. Belliotti points out, not only are there some interests of human beings that can be defeated after they die, but also there are some interests of human beings that can *only* be defeated after they die. He says:

> One's interests concerning the discharge of her will, the treatment of her corpse, and the maintenance of her reputation after she is dead can only be affected after she dies. So not only may humans have interests satisfiable after they are dead, but they have certain interests which are *only* satisfiable after they are dead.[49]

The above argument for the position that persons can be harmed by posthumous events can be expressed as follows:

(i) Some of a person's interests can survive the death of the person.
(ii) The interests which survive the death of the person may be impaired by posthumous events.

(iii) *Harm is the impairment of interest.*
(iv) Therefore, a person can be harmed by posthumous events.

Call this argument the 'interest-impairment theory *of posthumous harms*'.

In the last two sections, I have already shown that the death event can be a harm to a person. As I have emphasised before, if the death event is a harm to a person, then death (being dead) must be a harm to him as well.[50] Given this, it is therefore concluded that death (being dead) can also be a harm to a person. However, this position—death can be a harm—is also challenged by the missing subject problem which can be put thus:

(1) There cannot be any harm without a subject to be harmed.
(2) Death is the cessation of one's existence. At and after death, there is no subject.
(3) Given (2), there is no subject to be the subject of the harm of death.
(4) Therefore, death is not a harm.[51]

Call this the 'missing subject problem concerning the harm of death'.

To defend my position, it is necessary to locate the subject of the harm of death, when it is a harm. On the basis of the discussion of the missing subject problem concerning posthumous harms, I think that it is very easy to locate the subject of the harm of death, when it is a harm: *It is the ante-mortem person, whose interests are squelched, who is the subject of the harm of death.*

By the same token, the following conclusion can be reached: The subject of the harm of *premature death* is also the ante-mortem person. This provides a resolution of the missing subject problem.

Since I have located the subject of the harm of death (when it is a harm), the position that death can be a harm to the person who dies would be further secured. However, there is still a remaining difficulty with this conclusion.

If the subject of 'the harm of death' (or 'posthumous harms') is the *ante-mortem* person, then it would certainly imply that the subject *was* harmed by his own death (or by 'posthumous events') *before* his death. It is natural for some people, especially Epicureans, to ask:

How could an ante-mortem person be harmed by his own death *before* death? How could an ante-mortem person be harmed by something happening after his death? If an ante-mortem person could be harmed *at* or *after* his death by either his own death or posthumous events, then this would mean that an event at a later time could actually change a person's condition at an earlier time. If so, then 'the harm of death' and 'posthumous harms' are retroactive. This sounds odd.

However, in the next section, I will justify that it is really the case that the subject *was* harmed by his own death or by posthumous events *before* his death. This does not entail backward causation (i.e. no altering of the past). When we look at it more closely, it does not appear odd.[52]

4.4 THE TIMING OF THE HARM OF DEATH

In his paper, "A Solution to the Puzzle of When Death Harms Its Victims", Lamont claims that according to deprivation theorists there are three different views about the time at which the harm of death occurs: (1) Eternally, (2) Before Death, and (3) At No Time.[53] After considering these alternatives, Lamont claims that none of them is plausible. He argues that the most plausible view is 'At Death'.[54] I will now examine these four possible views in order.

Let us discuss the 'Eternal' view first. I will argue that Fred Feldman's 'Eternal' proposal cannot be counted as one of the alternatives, because this view is not in fact used by Feldman to answer the above question—When does the harm of death occur? In other words, Lamont has misunderstood Feldman.

In fact, with regard to this question, 'When does the harm of death occur?', Feldman adopts the same view as Lamont's—the 'At Death' proposal. Feldman says:

> Suppose a certain girl died in her youth. We are not concerned here about any puzzle about the date of her death. We may suppose we know that. Thus, in one sense, we know precisely when the misfortune occurred.[55]

On the other hand, I claim that the 'Eternal' proposal is used by Feldman to express the following notion:

> The harm of someone's (P's) death is a fact. This fact is timeless. That is, it not only exists at the time when the harm occurs, but it also exists in the present, the future, and even the past. This is just like the case 'Caesar died in 44 BC'. Once 'Caesar died in 44 BC' is a fact, that fact is not only true in 44 BC, but also true in the present, the past (before 44 BC), and the future. (I will not discuss here whether facts can exist eternally or not).

This claim can be supported by Feldman's statement on the 'Eternal' proposal:

> The present question is, rather, a question about when her death is a misfortune for her. If Lindsay is the girl, and d is the state of affairs of Lindsay dying on December 7, 1987, then the question is this: 'Precisely when is d bad for Lindsay?'…So our question comes to this: 'Precisely when is it the case that the value for Lindsay of the nearest world in which d occurs is lower than the value for her of the nearest world in which d does not occur?'[56]

Unfortunately, Lamont mistakes Feldman's question, 'When does the fact of the harm of P's death obtain? (i.e. When is the fact of the harm of P's death true?)' for 'When does the harm of P's death happen?' Because of this, Lamont comments, '…his [Feldman's] analysis of when the harm of death occurs is problematic.'[57]

In short, the 'Eternal' proposal is not a view propounded by Feldman to answer the question, 'When does the harm of death happen?'

In fact, there are two different interpretations of 'When does the harm of death happen?' These will be discussed below.

Let us now move on to the 'At No Time' proposal. On a sympathetic reading, Nagel seems to try to distinguish two notions: (1) the suffering of a misfortune by someone (P), and (2) the misfortune itself. Nagel, by using this distinction, wants to argue that P is a concrete individual, so P has a spatio-temporal location. However, misfortune (or harm) is an abstract idea or some kind of relationship, so it is impossible for it to be located in space or time. In other words, it is possible for P to be harmed at a certain time, possible, that is, to know when P's suffering the harm occurs. However, it is impossible to know when the harm itself happens (i.e. there is no time at which the harm itself occurs).

This point is implicitly expressed by Nagel as follows:

Although the spatial and temporal locations of the individual who suffered the loss are clear enough, the misfortune itself cannot be so easily located...he must have existence and specific spatial and temporal location even if the loss itself does not.[58]

Regardless, Nagel does not disagree that P can be harmed at a certain time. Thus, to the question, 'When does P's being harmed by death happen?', it is possible for Nagel to adopt the 'At Death' proposal as well. On the other hand, to the other question, 'When does the harm itself happen?', Nagel will answer, 'At no time' (I will not discuss here whether the harm itself is timeless).

I believe that we should read 'When does the harm of P's death happen?' as 'When does P's being harmed by death happen?', rather than 'When does the harm itself happen?' In this way we can avoid Nagel's ontological difficulty. There is no doubt that this question, 'When does P's being harmed by death happen?' is the real 'when' question philosophers have found puzzling in the case of death. However, even if 'When does P's being harmed by death happen?' is the same question as 'When does the harm itself happen?', it is harmless for us just to use the first question for discussing the timing.

To show the problem with Nagel's 'At No Time' proposal, Lamont asks us to consider the following two situations.

Suppose Alf the anaesthetist deliberately administers an overdose of anaesthesia to Betty. It immediately causes her severe brain damage, turning her from a competent adult into a happy person with the mind of a two year old. Betty, however, in no way suffers as a result of this procedure or afterwards—the harm is purely relational, not experiential.[59]

In this case Lamont supposes that Alf argues in his defence that there is no time at which he harmed Betty. According to Lamont, 'we would not want to accept such a defence, but how could somebody supporting the At No Time proposal block it?'[60]

Nagel can reply, "According to the 'At No Time' proposal, it is true that there is no time at which the harm itself occurs. However, it is not true that there is no time at which Alf harmed Betty."

Another case is, 'Henry, who is also a Nagel scholar...lops off Catherine's head with his sword.'[61]

With regard to this case, Lamont writes:

> He [Nagel] needs an argument to block the implication that if there
> is no time at which Henry's victim is harmed, then there is no time at
> which Henry harmed his victim…Henry can claim there is no time at
> which his victim was harmed.[62]

Again Nagel can reply, "According to the 'At No Time' proposal, there is no
implication that there is no time at which Henry's victim is harmed."
Furthermore, he might say, 'Catherine is harmed just at the time when Henry
lops off her head (i.e. when she dies).'

In short, the 'At No Time' proposal is not the view used by Nagel to
answer the question, 'When does P's being harmed by death happen?'

Now, the alternatives are only the 'At Death' proposal and the 'Before
Death' proposal.

Let us discuss the 'At Death' proposal first. Concerning the question,
'Who is the subject of harm by death?' both the 'At Death' proposal and the
'Before Death' proposal say that it is the 'ante-mortem person'.[63] This is
right, because posthumous people cannot be the subjects of any interests or
harms. However, they give very different interpretations of 'ante-mortem
person'. This partly accounts for the difference in the two proposals.

Suppose P was born at T_0 and died at T_1. Feinberg and Pitcher stipulate:

(1) There exists the living, breathing P between T_0 and T_1 (but not
    including T_1).
(2) From T_1 on, there is only a dead P in whatever form (e.g. a
    corpse).[64]

However, Lamont believes: (i) there exists the living, breathing P between T_0
and T_1 (but not including T_1), and (ii) from T_1 on there is in addition to a dead
P an ante-mortem P.[65]

Lamont asserts that the living and breathing P is not the subject of harm by
death, because 'no such person exists at death.'[66] On the other hand, he
claims, it is the ante-mortem person (at T_1) that is the subject of harm by
death.

However, the notion of a person at death (and thereafter) is problematic.
Lamont gives no metaphysical explanation to support this notion. That is to
say, he does not explain how it is possible there is still an ante-mortem person
after someone's death. Conversely, this notion simply conflicts with his own

assumption: 'It will be assumed throughout that a consequence of death is that the person no longer exists, i.e. the person does not continue in some other form.'[67] The ante-mortem person at death and thereafter is supposed by Lamont to be the subject of posthumous harms (and harm by death). However, since P does not exist in any form at death and after, there is no real subject of posthumous harms (and harm by death) in Lamont's 'At Death' proposal. In a word, the 'At Death' proposal is compromised and should therefore be rejected.

In fact, the question, 'When does the harm event of death happen?' is very different from the question, 'When does P's being harmed by death happen?' By adopting an ambiguous formulation 'When does the harm of death to P happen?', Lamont conflates these two questions. Lamont is correct when he says that the harm of death to P happens at P's death, if 'When does the harm of death to P happen?' is interpreted as 'When does the harm event of death happen?' Death as a harm event occurs at the time of death. However, he is not correct to make the same statement, if 'When does the harm of death to P happen?' is interpreted as 'When does P's being harmed by death happen?' And it is this latter question 'When does P's being harmed by death happen?' which is the question that many philosophers have found puzzling.

The difference between these two questions can be illustrated more clearly in cases of posthumous harms. In such cases, the 'At Death' proposal yields unwelcome results. Suppose that Q spreads a false and malicious rumour about P after P's death. Since P has an interest in his posthumous good reputation, P is harmed by the rumour. Here, the harm event (Q's spreading the rumour) and P's being harmed are two separate things. Lamont accepts that Q harms P when he spreads the rumour at T_2. However, since P no longer exists at T_2, how could he be harmed at T_2?

The last view to consider is the 'Before Death' proposal. I believe that this is the most reasonable of the four views.

Lamont's account makes use of a distinction between hard and soft facts which can be explained as follows. A fact is a soft fact about T_1 insofar as its obtaining at T_1 depends on some fact obtaining at a later time T_2; whereas a hard fact does not. For example, 'John wakes up at eight' is a hard fact about eight o'clock, because it does not depend on any state of affairs which obtains after eight. On the other hand, 'At eight John wakes up four hours prior to eating lunch' is a soft fact about eight o'clock, because it depends on a fact, 'John eats lunch' which obtains at noon.[68]

By making use of the soft/hard fact distinction, Lamont tries to refute Feinberg's 'Before Death' proposal. He argues:

(1) What Feinberg's 'Before Death' proposal claims about the timing of the harm of death is a soft fact claim.

(2) But this soft fact claim is not the type of answer that philosophers have been looking for when discussing the puzzle of the timing of the harm of death.

(3) Therefore, Feinberg's 'Before Death' proposal is not satisfactory.[69]

Concerning (2), Lamont does not give any further explanation. That is to say, he does not justify his claim that the soft fact about the timing of death does not provide the right answer to the puzzle about the timing of the harm of death. I believe that the soft/hard fact distinction does not help to resolve the issue of the timing of the harm of death. When discussing the timing of the harm of death, is there any essential difference between the following two facts about the past?

(i) Caesar was harmed by death in 44 BC—(hard fact).

(ii) Caesar was harmed by death 2029 years prior to Fischer's writing his paper 'L' in 1985—(soft fact).

In terms of the timing of the harm of death, (ii) is based on just the same fact about the past that (i) is. That is, although the soft/hard fact distinction is important in debates about God's foreknowledge and human freedom, it is not relevant for the timing of the harm of death.

On the other hand, I believe that what really matters about the issue of the timing of the harm of death is a potential/actual fact distinction. That is to say, when discussing the puzzle of the timing of the harm of death, it is important to distinguish between the fact which actually happens (which may be expressed as either a hard fact or a soft fact), and the potential (or possible) fact which has not happened yet. In other words, it is a necessary condition for the 'Before Death' view to be the case that the 'Before Death' view does not apply to the potential fact.

By using the hard/soft fact distinction, Lamont attempts to show that:

(1) Feinberg's 'Before Death' proposal about the timing of the harm of death is a potential fact claim (in Lamont's words, an 'open question').

(2) This will lead to some awkward or even implausible and misleading results.[70]

Thus, it is better, when discussing the timing of the harm of death, to give up using the hard/soft fact distinction, noting that its exact characterisation is still problematic. [71] Instead, it is more useful in this instance to adopt the potential/actual fact distinction.

Let us examine whether Feinberg's 'Before Death' proposal is a claim about a potential fact or not.

It is true that Feinberg does not avoid applying his theory to potential facts. This can be found from an example of Pitcher's which he uses:

> If the world should be blasted to smithereens during the next presidency after Ronald Reagan's, this would make it true (be responsible for the fact) that even now, during Reagan's term, he is the penultimate president of the United States. [72]

Feinberg adds:

> Similarly, the financial collapse of the life-insurance company through which I have protected my loved dependants, occurring, let us imagine, five minutes after my death, several years in the future, makes it true that my present interest in my children's security is harmed, and therefore, that I am harmed too, though I know it not. [73]

In the former case, the situation Feinberg describes is a hypothetical condition. It is still possible that the disaster will not happen. Similarly, in the latter case, it is possible that the life-insurance company will not collapse. Even if the company does collapse, it does not imply that my children will definitely be harmed. In brief, the facts mentioned by Feinberg here are only potential (or possible) facts.

However, if this theory can be modified to avoid applying to the potential facts (i.e. the modified 'Before Death' theory applies only to the actual facts), then it will be a reasonable proposal to answer the timing question, 'When does P's being harmed by death occur?'

Let me illustrate the modified 'Before Death' theory by the following example:

> There is a soccer game. Both M and N are in the same team. M made a very good pass to N at T_1—the ball was just in front of the net and the other team's keeper and players were all away from the net. M had set up a very good chance for getting a goal. What was

needed was an appropriate kick from N which is very easy for N. N kicked the ball into the net at T_2.

It is not correct to claim at the time before T_2 that M had made a significant contribution to the score. The reason simply is that at that time T_1 they had not scored yet. It is still possible for N to miss the good chance. Only after T_2, can we correctly claim that M had made a significant contribution in obtaining a point. Before T_2, the claim 'M made a significant contribution at T_1' is about a potential (or very possible) fact. While, at and after T_2, the claim is about an actual (or real) fact. In a sense, N's kicking the ball at T_2 made M's contribution for one point true. In other words, before T_2, what M made was only a potential (or possible) contribution. N's kicking the ball made this potential (or possible) contribution into an actual (or real) one. That is to say, in order to become an actual contribution, what M made still needs to rely on another agent or event. In short, it is in the sense of actual fact that the modified 'Before Death' theorist claims that P suffers a harm from death before death. That is, the modified 'Before Death' theorist claims it after P's death. P's death is a potential harm throughout P's life time which is realised or actualised at the moment of death.

Now let us explain, by using the modified 'Before Death' theory, the following case Lamont offers, 'Suppose...Andrew at T_1 has an interest in being alive and seeing some event at T_3. Suppose it is now T_3 and, as it turned out, Andrew died at T_2.'[74]

In this case, before T_2 the claim 'the interest that Andrew had at T_1 was going to be thwarted' is a potential fact about T_1. However, at T_2 and after, the same claim is an actual fact. At T_3, not only can we state the exact time at which he has an interest in being alive and seeing some event at T_3 (i.e. T_1), but we can also point out the exact time when Andrew died (i.e. T_2). In any case, both of these two events are facts and cannot be changed.

Lamont raises the following objection to refute Feinberg's 'Before Death' view:

> Making such a claim [that the interest that Andrew had at T_1 was going to be thwarted] involves saying a person is harmed by her death when the question of the time and even fact of her death is an open one. While it may simply be awkward in the determinism /fatalism case to claim of people wandering around the streets that they are currently harmed by their deaths it is mistaken to claim it in non-deterministic/non-fatalistic worlds. Whether these people have

any interests that will be thwarted is an open question, either because they will not die or because, when their death comes, it does not thwart any of their interests. If this is open, then the timing of the harm of their deaths should also be open...*it is open whether death will harm people when it happens*, it is open when they will die, and it is even open whether they will die at all.[75] (My emphasis.)

In fact, Lamont has successfully challenged Feinberg's view here. However, the modified 'Before Death' theorist can easily reply to this challenge as follows.

It is clear that the claim Lamont mentions above is made before T_2. With regard to this claim, Lamont's comment is correct. That is, before these people die, the following are all true:

(1) Whether they have any interests that will be thwarted is an open question.
(2) Whether death will harm people when it happens is open.
(3) When they will die is open.
(4) Whether they will die is open.

In short, this claim is only about a potential fact. I think the modified 'Before Death' theorist agrees with Lamont on this point. However, at and after the time when these people die, it is also true that all these questions become actual ones. That is, this claim is then about an actual fact. It is the latter claim that the modified 'Before Death' theorist means in saying that 'the interest that Andrew had at T_1 was going to be thwarted'. Therefore, I conclude that Lamont does not successfully refute the 'Before Death' proposal.

As for Lamont's other objection, '...the Before Death answer is not satisfactory. A view that involves the very counterintuitive claim that a murderer harmed his victim twenty years (or whatever) before he killed her...'[76] This sounds odd only because Lamont conflates the harm event and P's being harmed. The harm event occurs when the murder took place, but P's being harmed can occur at an earlier time, i.e. *before* he was murdered, *before* his death. This is no longer counterintuitive.

According to all the above discussions, I conclude that the 'Before Death' view is the correct answer to the question, 'When does someone's (P's) being harmed by death occur?'[77]

Since I have shown the timing of someone's (P's) being harmed by his own death (and posthumous events)—*before death*, the claim that '*death can be a harm to the person who dies*'[78] is once again vindicated.[79]

CHAPTER FIVE

The Lucretian Symmetry Argument

In this chapter, I will reject the Lucretian symmetry argument by criticising some proposals from recent philosophers. To achieve this, let me explicate the Lucretian symmetry argument first.

5.1 EXPLICATION OF THE LUCRETIAN SYMMETRY ARGUMENT

Joining his master, Epicurus, in the campaign against the fear of death, Lucretius[1] poses a famous and now much-discussed symmetry argument—the Lucretian symmetry argument. This argument, if correct, would lead to the conclusion—*death is not a harm, so we should not fear our death*. This conclusion directly challenges my conclusion reached in Chapter Four— *death can be a harm to the person who dies*. In order to defend my position, it is necessary to reject the Lucretian symmetry argument. To reject the Lucretian symmetry argument, it is important to examine it in detail, as follows.

In his *On the Nature of Things*, Lucretius says:

> Think too how the bygone antiquity of everlasting time before our birth was nothing to us. Nature holds this up to us as a mirror of the time yet to come after our death. Is there anything in this that looks appalling, anything that wears an aspect of gloom? Is it not more untroubled than any sleep?[2]

Call this the 'Lucretian symmetry argument'.

Put simply, the main point of this argument is:

> Our future nonexistence and our past nonexistence are *equally* devoid of value for us now. And the fact that our past nonexistence is devoid of value explains why it is irrational to be presently concerned about our past nonexistence. Therefore, it is irrational to be presently concerned about the future state of being dead.[3]

This argument has been appropriately reconstructed by Rosenbaum as follows:

> (1) No one fears the time before which one existed.
> (2) The time before which one existed is relevantly like one's future nonexistence (in that one cannot be affected negatively in either period). (This is the 'symmetry thesis.')
> (3) It is reasonable for one to fear something relevantly like what one does not fear only if one justifiably believes that the two things are relevantly different.
> (4) No one justifiably believes that one's future nonexistence is relevantly different from one's past nonexistence.
> THEREFORE, it is not reasonable now for one to fear one's future nonexistence, one's being dead, one's death.[4]

Call this argument the 'standard interpretation of the Lucretian symmetry argument'.

For a more effective discussion of the Lucretian symmetry argument (and its standard interpretation), let me explicate it in more detail.

Firstly, the starting point of the Lucretian symmetry argument (and its standard interpretation) is that we, as normal and reasonably rational persons, are indifferent (or nearly indifferent) to our prenatal nonexistence. Indeed, no one really fears one's past nonexistence. Since this is a fact, both Lucretians and anti-Lucretians should accept it. But note that the attitude toward to the time before our birth (or after our death) is one thing, and the value-evaluation of this period (i.e. deciding whether this period is bad or not) is another. As Williams quite correctly points out, considering whether death (or prenatal nonexistence) can reasonably be regarded as an evil is not the same as considering whether death (or prenatal nonexistence) should be feared.[5]

Secondly, it is assumed that in the Lucretian symmetry argument, Lucretius directs his attention to the fear of nonbeing or ceasing to be, but not to the fears of (painful) dying, or the unknown.[6]

Thirdly, the Lucretian symmetry argument (and its standard interpretation) apparently endeavours to prove the following conclusions:

> (i) Neither prenatal nonexistence nor death is a harm.
> (ii) It is not reasonable now for us to fear either our prenatal nonexistence or our death.

Here, (i) has theoretical priority over (ii). For *only if* we make sure whether prenatal nonexistence is a harm and whether death is a harm, can we properly consider the appropriate attitudes toward these two periods. That is, the 'symmetry thesis' is the crucial premise in the Lucretian symmetry argument (and its standard interpretation). To refute the Lucretian *symmetry* argument, it is better and easier for us to focus on (i)—the symmetry thesis—rather than (ii). In so doing, logically speaking, there are three possible approaches to rejecting the Luretian symmetry argument:

> (1) Showing that prenatal nonexistence is a harm, but death is not a harm.
> (2) Showing that both prenatal nonexistence and death are harms.
> (3) Showing that prenatal nonexistence is not a harm, but death is a harm.[7]

These three approaches can be called: (i) Prenatal harm approach, (ii) Prenatal-and-Posthumous harm approach, (iii) Posthumous harm approach. In the next section, I will discuss them in order.

5.2 THE FAILURE OF THE LUCRETIAN SYMMETRY ARGUMENT

The Prenatal harm approach, Prenatal-and-Posthumous harm approach, and Posthumous harm approach are adopted by various recent philosophers. Let us now examine these three approaches.

I. Prenatal Harm Approach

Walter Glannon suggests a temporal asymmetry to the effect that *prenatal nonexistence is a harm but death is not a harm.*[8] In proposing this view, Glannon adopts the Existence Requirement. He states, 'I have been appealing to the Existence Requirement…to ground my own argument.'[9]

The Existence Requirement is understood by Glannon as: 'A person can be the subject of some misfortune [or harm] *only if* he exists at the time the misfortune [or harm] occurs.'[10] (My emphasis.)

Furthermore, Glannon explicates the Existence Requirement as follows:

> On the intuitively plausible assumption that the *value* of our lives is a function of what we *can* experience, something is… good or bad for us *only if* it is possible for us actually to experience it as such.[11] (My emphasis.)

On the basis of the Existence Requirement, Glannon argues that death is not a harm because it cannot affect the experienced quality of our lives. Therefore death should not be an object of our rational concern.[12]

Conversely, Glannon argues that prenatal nonexistence is a harm since it may function as causes bringing about temporally remote effects that can make a significant difference to the experienced quality of our lives. Therefore, prenatal nonexistence may be an object of our rational concern.[13] Glanon offers the following examples to support his view:

> A human organism begins to exist when the father's sperm fertilizes the mother's egg to form the zygote from which the organism develops into a person. Prior to conception, exposure to an occupational or environmental carcinogen can damage the father's sperm, which may manifest itself in some disease or handicap in his child and in turn have the effect of limiting that person's prospects for enjoying goods over the course of her lifespan. Furthermore, during the prenatal period when one exists *in utero*, a pregnant woman may contract a viral infection like rubella, which can cause blindness, deafness, or a congenital heart disorder in the child. In addition, daughters of women who received the drug DES (diethylstilbesterol) to prevent premature labor during pregnancy may suffer, after reaching sexual maturity, from such effects as malformed reproductive tracts, infertility, and vaginal cancer. Also,

people born immediately after an influenza epidemic may be at significantly higher risk for developing schizophrenia as adults than babies born in years without high flu rates. Or consider such genetically heritable diseases as cystic fibrosis and Huntington's chorea, whose causes in the parents' genes exist long before the birth of those who must suffer from their effects both in childhood and adulthood.[14]

Glannon concludes his above discussion with the following argument:

(1) It is rational for one to be concerned now about something relevantly like what one is not concerned about only if one justifiably believes that the two are relevantly different.

(2) Past nonexistence is relevantly different from future nonexistence insofar as states of affairs that obtain during the former period can affect persons adversely in respects in which states of affairs obtaining during the latter period cannot (asymmetry thesis).

(3) One is justified in believing that past nonexistence is relevantly different from future nonexistence.

(4) It is rational to be concerned now about what can actually affect a person adversely.

(5) Therefore, although it is not rational for one to be concerned now about one's future nonexistence, it may be rational for one to be concerned now about one's past nonexistence.[15]

I think that Glannon's proposal is simply incorrect. Firstly, Glannon argues: Prenatal nonexistence is a harm since some prenatal events may function as causes bringing about a harm to us. However, it is also the case that some prenatal events may function as causes bringing about a benefit to us. Consider the following case:

John is a very successful lawyer in New York City. He is rich, knowledgeable, and respectable. Most importantly, he is very satisfied with his life. Before he was born, for some reason his parents were allowed to move to New York City from a very poor village in Africa. People in that village do not even have enough food to eat. Of course, most of them (including his cousins) cannot afford to go to school.

In this case, this event (i.e. John's parents's moving to New York City) may have done a great benefit to him. Thus, it is not clear whether, overall, prenatal events may function as causes bringing a harm to us.

Even if prenatal events may, overall, function as causes bringing a harm to us, it does not follow that prenatal nonexistence is a harm to us. The reason is as follows.

The notion 'the harm of prenatal nonexistence' and the notion 'prenatal harms' are different. Similarly, the notion 'the harm of posthumous nonexistence (i.e. death)' is different from the notion 'posthumous harms'. In any case, prenatal nonexistence is a state located in an everlasting time before our birth. Some events occurring in this state may function as causes bringing about a harm to us. However, it does not therefore follow that the state which these events are in is a harm to us. In short, there is at least a gap between 'prenatal events may function as causes bringing about a harm to us' and 'prenatal nonexistence is a harm to us'. Therefore, Glannon fails to reject Lucretius' view that prenatal nonexistence is not a harm to us. Indeed, prenatal nonexistence is not a harm to us, as will be shown below.

In addition, according to Glannon's proposal, posthumous harms cannot be real. For any events happening after one dies may not bring about any effects that can make a significant difference to the actually *experienced* quality of one's life. However, in Chapter Four, Section Three, I have shown that persons *can* be harmed by posthumous events.

I think the reason why Glannon's proposal entails this incorrect conclusion—posthumous harms cannot be real—is: *His proposal has essentially relied on the Existence Requirement which is incorrect.* Indeed, we can easily find situations in which something is regarded as a harm or misfortune for a person, but cannot (logically or metaphysically) be experienced by him. For example, when someone's life work has come to nothing after he dies, most people would think that he has suffered a misfortune. In short, the Existence Requirement, as has been shown in Chapter One, Section Two, is incorrect, so Glannon's proposal should not be accepted.

Let us now move on to the Prenatal-and-Posthumous harm approach.

II. Prenatal-and-Posthumous Harm Approach

The most widespread theory for explaining why death is a harm is the deprivation theory.[16] According to this theory, death is the deprivation of the good things of life. That is, when life is, on balance, good, then death is bad insofar as it robs one of this good: if one had died later than one actually did, then one would have had more of the good things of life.[17]

To the deprivation theory, Lucretians might pose the following challenge:

> It seems that prenatal nonexistence constitutes a deprivation in a sense analogous to that in which death is a deprivation: if a person had been born earlier than he actually was born, then he would have had more of the good things in life. After all, being born at the time at which one was born (rather than earlier) is a deprivation in the same sense as dying at the time when one dies (rather than later). Therefore, if death, according to the deprivation theory, is a harm, then, by the same token, prenatal nonexistence must be a harm as well.[18]

To this challenge, some deprivation theorists might answer, 'Yes, prenatal nonexistence is a harm as well.' Apparently, their position, if true, would render the Lucretian symmetry argument unsound. Because of this, Lucretians might raise another challenge:

> If prenatal nonexistence is a harm, why do we treat it with indifference? That is to say, why should we treat prenatal and posthumous nonexistence asymmetrically, given they are value symmetrical?

With regard to this challenge, Parfit offers a response. Parfit's proposal can be briefly put as follows:

> We have a (not irrational) bias toward the future to the extent that there are cases where we are indifferent toward our own past suffering but *not* indifferent toward our own future suffering. Since there are such cases, and the attitudes therein seem rational, the general principle that it is always rational to have symmetric attitudes toward (comparable) past and future bads is false, and so it might be true that it is not irrational to have asymmetric attitudes toward our own past and future nonexistence (where such periods of nonexistence are taken to be *bads*). Thus, death could be considered a bad thing for us, and yet we need not assume symmetric attitudes toward death and prenatal nonexistence.[19]

In his much-discussed analysis of attitude asymmetry in *Reasons and Persons*, Parfit uses the following example to support his above position:

> I am in some hospital to have some kind of surgery. Since this is completely safe, and always successful, I have no fears about the effects. The surgery may be brief, or it may instead take a long time. Because I have to co-operate with the surgeon, I cannot have anaesthetics. I have had this surgery once before, and I can remember how painful it is. Under a new policy, because the operation is so painful, patients are now afterwards made to forget it. Some drug removes their memories of the last few hours.
>
> I have just woken up. I cannot remember going to sleep. I ask my nurse if it has been decided when my operation is to be, and how long it must take. She says that she knows the facts about both me and another patient, but that she cannot remember which facts apply to whom. She can tell me only that the following is true. I may be the patient who had his operation yesterday. In that case, my operation was the longest ever performed, lasting ten hours. I may instead be the patient who is to have a short operation later today. It is either true that I did suffer for ten hours, or true that I shall suffer for one hour.
>
> I ask the nurse to find out which is true. While she is away, it is clear to me which I prefer to be true. If I learn that the first is true, I shall be greatly relieved.[20]

I think that Parfit's proposal is problematic. The main problem with his proposal is that, as Anthony L. Brueckner and John Martin Fischer suggest, 'Parfit's case involves a bad for a person that is *experienced as bad by the person*...But death is not a bad of this kind.'[21]

Although we *might* have a bias, as Parfit suggests, toward future *experienced* bads (or harms), this bias does not seem to be applicable to bads (or harms) of which we are never aware or which we do not experience consciously. Indeed, cases that are structurally similar to Parfit's except involving bads (or harms) not experienced as bad by the person yield *symmetric* attitudes. To show this, Rosenbaum offers the following example:

> Suppose that being secretly hated by someone could be bad for a person. The hatred might affect the person, but in ways of which the person would never become aware. It is not at all plausible that one

would be more anxious about the future occurrence of this bad than one would be about its past occurrence.[22]

Even worse, in certain circumstances, we can have bias toward *past* bads (or harms), but not *future* bads (or harms). With relation to this, Rosenbaum says:

> There are bads [or harms] which most persons would prefer in their *futures* rather than in their pasts. Consider the loss of one's reputation. Most persons would prefer that this bad [or harm] be in their *futures* instead of in their pasts. Perhaps the reason for this is that the loss of one's reputation can have far-reaching effects on one, effects that reach into the future. The preference may be due to the fact that persons would like to minimize the effects of some such bad [or harm], and the effects might be less if the bad [or harm] occurred in the future, closer to the end of one's life.[23]

Apparently, one's death, if a harm at all, is not the sort of harm which a person could experience consciously or be aware of. Therefore, Parfit's version of the bias toward the future (experienced) bads (or harms) cannot apply to such alleged bads (or harms) as death.

In the face of the difficulty Parfit encounters, Brueckner and Fischer modify Parfit's proposal. Instead of adopting Parfit's version of future bias, they take another temporal bias—we have a temporal asymmetry in our attitudes toward 'experienced goods'. That is, Brueckner and Fischer believe that we are indifferent to past experienced pleasures but look forward to future experienced pleasures.[24] To support this, they offer the following variant of Parfit's example:

> Imagine that you are in some hospital to test a drug. The drug induces intense pleasure for an hour followed by amnesia. You awaken and ask the nurse about your situation. She says that either you tried the drug yesterday (and had an hour of pleasure) or you will try the drug tomorrow (and will have an hour of pleasure). While she checks on your status, it is clear that you prefer to have the pleasure tomorrow.[25]

By making use of the temporal asymmetry in our attitudes toward *experienced goods*, Brueckner and Fischer claim:

Death is a bad [or a harm] insofar as it is a deprivation of the good things in life (some of which, let us suppose, are 'experienced as good' by the individual). If death occurs in the future, then it is a deprivation of something to which we look forward and about which we care—*future experienced goods*. But prenatal nonexistence is a deprivation of *past experienced goods*, goods to which we are indifferent. Death deprives us of something we care about, whereas prenatal nonexistence deprives us of something to which we are indifferent.[26](My emphasis.)

With this, they conclude:

Thus we can defend Nagel's account of the badness of death [i.e. the deprivation theory] by explaining the asymmetry in our *attitudes* toward prenatal and posthumous nonexistence.[27] (My emphasis.)

Accordingly, it is natural for us to think that Brueckner and Fischer intend to defend the Prenatal-and-Posthumous harm approach by modifying Parfit's version of temporal bias. That is to say, they, like Parfit, take the position: *Both prenatal nonexistence and death are harms. But, we are indifferent to our prenatal nonexistence although we do care about our own deaths.*[28] Surprisingly, they want more. After offering the above analysis and suggestion, they emphatically conclude:

If we have asymmetric *attitudes* toward past and future experienced goods, then *death is a bad thing in a way in which prenatal nonexistence is not.*[29] (My emphasis.)

Accordingly, Brueckner and Fischer's proposal can be expressed as follows:

(1) Since our asymmetric attitudes toward past and future experienced goods seem *rational*, the general principle that it is always rational to have symmetric attitudes toward (comparable) past and future experienced goods is false.

(2) If so, it may well be *rational* to have asymmetric attitudes toward our own past and future nonexistence: death deprives us of something we care about whereas prenatal nonexistence deprives us of something to which we are indifferent.

(3) Therefore, if we have *rational* asymmetric attitudes toward past and future experienced goods, then death is a bad thing in a way in which prenatal nonexistence is not.[30]

With regard to Brueckner and Fischer's proposal, Ishtiyaque Haji comments as follows:

> Suppose Brueckner and Fischer are right about the asymmetry in our attitudes toward past and future experienced goods. Still, this alleged fact about attitudinal asymmetry could not be used to corroborate the *asymmetry thesis* that whereas a person's post-vital times are bad for him, his pre-vital times are not.[31]

Indeed, the conclusion of Brueckner and Fischer's above argument (and thus their proposal) is problematic. I will now raise three difficulties for premise (3) in the above argument, and, thus, for their proposal.

(I). According to the deprivation theory, death is a bad (or a harm) since it is the deprivation of the goods of life. Clearly, the deprivation theory has presupposed that *the deprivation of goods is a bad (or a harm)*. If we accept the deprivation theory and also believe that prenatal nonexistence is the deprivation of the goods of life, then, in virtue of the presupposition of the deprivation theory, we should concede that prenatal nonexistence (or not being born earlier) is a harm as well.[32]

Apparently, in their discussion about this issue, Brueckner and Fischer *do* accept the deprivation theory. In their paper "The Asymmetry of Early Death and Late Birth", they say: 'We attempted to defend *the deprivation thesis* by arguing for a specific and limited asymmetry claim.'[33] (My emphasis.)

Besides, they also believe that prenatal nonexistence is the deprivation of the goods of life. In their another paper "Why is Death Bad?", they say: 'Death is a bad insofar as it is a deprivation of...future experienced goods...[whereas] *prenatal nonexistence is a deprivation of past experienced goods...*'[34] (My emphasis.)

Therefore, Brueckner and Fischer should at least concede that prenatal nonexistence (or not being born earlier) is a harm *in a common sense*.

(II). 'Rational' is an ambiguous term. It might sometimes be very easily confused with 'reasonable'. To avoid possible confusion in our later discussion, I suggest that the term 'rational' in Brueckner and Fischer's above argument may be understood as 'psychologically acceptable'.

Suppose our bias toward the future *experienced* goods is 'psychologically acceptable', then, apparently, it is a psychological fact. Here, Brueckner and Fischer can be challenged as follows:

> Why should the mere particular psychological fact change the value of prenatal nonexistence? After all, the claim that our prenatal times are bad for us is directly derived from the deprivation theory and the belief that prenatal nonexistence is the deprivation of the goods of life, both of which are accepted by Brueckner and Fischer. Unless they can raise enough reasons for this change, it is invalid for Brueckner and Fischer to conclude that prenatal nonexistence is not a bad thing. That is to say, without a suitable non-question begging principle that bridges the gap between 'it is rational for S to care about his posthumous nonexistence (i.e. death) whereas indifferent to his prenatal nonexistence' to 'whereas S's posthumous non-existence is a bad thing for S, S's prenatal nonexistence is not', Brueckner and Fischer cannot defend their position.[35]

The reason Brueckner and Fischer actually give for this bridge is: It is in general *rational* to have asymmetric attitudes to past and future good experiences. If this is indeed a fact, then it is reasonable to think that death is a bad thing in a way in which prenatal nonexistence is not.[36]

In defending their position against Haji's attack, Brueckner and Fischer revise their above point as:

> If it is true that it is *rational* for a person to prefer his pleasurable experiences in the future rather than the past, given that the total number of such experiences is held fixed, then it is plausible to suppose that posthumous nonexistence is a bad thing for a person in a way in which prenatal nonexistence is not.[37] (My emphasis.)

In short, the main point they use for supporting their position is, '...value comes not simply from having certain attitudes but from the *rationality* of those attitudes.'[38] (My emphasis.)

But, what is really the reason for Brueckner and Fischer to conclude that death is a bad thing in a way in which prenatal nonexistence is not? Even if taking this revised point, why values can come from the *rationality* of attitudes? Disappointingly, throughout their three relevant papers, "Why Is Death Bad" , "Death's Badness", and "The Asymmetry of Early Death and Late Birth", Brueckner and Fischer do *not* give any further explanation. Without some further acceptable explanation, Brueckner and Fischer are implicitly begging the question in their adoption of the principle that *values can come from rational attitudes.*

If this principle is problematic, then the conclusion derived from this principle—*prenatal nonexistence is not a bad thing*—is doubtful as well. Given this, their position that *death is a bad thing in a way in which prenatal nonexistence is not* is also problematic.

(III). Perhaps Brueckner and Fischer can find a way out by adopting a particular axiology—subjectivism. [39] Subjectivism and objectivism are understood by Haji as follows:

> According to subjectivist theories, states of affairs have value only in relation to the affections of persons. The value of a state of affairs for a person…is identical to the value, if any, that that state of affairs has for that person. A state of affairs, S1…has value for a person, P, if and only if P has the relevant 'affective attitude' toward to S1…In contrast, the distinguishing feature of objectivist theories is the denial of [subjectivist theories]. States of affairs, according to objectivists, have value independently of being desired, or preferred, or cared for, by anyone. [40]

By using this subjectivism, Brueckner and Fischer may argue for their position as follows:

> That some states of affairs have value in relation to us is only in virtue of the fact that we care for them. If we care for certain future states of affairs (e.g. death), those states of affair *can* be good or bad for us, depending on the situation. If we are indifferent toward past states of affairs (e.g. prenatal nonexistence), those states of affairs are axiologically neutral for us.[41]

However, in their paper "Death's Badness", Brueckner and Fischer clearly reject subjectivism. They say:

Indeed, despite the appearance engendered by some uncareful formulations, we wish to reject *subjectivism*. Our view is that *value does not come from an individual's actually caring about something...*[42] (My emphasis.)

Because of their rejection of *subjectivism* (i.e. adopting objectivism), Brueckner and Fischer face more difficulties. Let me explain.

The principle Brueckner and Fischer use to justify their position is: *Values can come from rational attitudes.* Either this principle is correct or it is incorrect. If this principle is incorrect, then, according to my analysis in (I), apparently Brueckner and Fischer should concede that prenatal nonexistence is a harm although it is always *rational* to be indifferent to past experienced goods. On the other hand, even if this principle is correct (which is very unlikely), it is still implausible for Brueckner and Fischer to claim that prenatal nonexistence is not a harm. The reason for this is the following.

As shown above, Brueckner and Fischer adopt the deprivation theory and also believe that prenatal nonexistence is the deprivation of the goods of life. Given this, according to the discussion in (I), they should at least concede that prenatal nonexistence is a harm *in a common sense*. Now, suppose it is the case that *values can come from rational attitudes.* Then, it appears that there can be two different kinds of bads (or harms) here: (i) bads (or harms) *in a common sense*, and (ii) bads (or harms) *in an attitude sense*. In other words, prenatal nonexistence is *bad in a common sense*, whereas it is *not bad in an attitude sense*. Now, the question here is: 'Given the deprivation theory, which sense should we take when we evaluate the value of prenatal nonexistence, (i) or (ii)?' To sort out this question, it is helpful to consider the case of the evaluation of death. Suppose we are the deprivation theorists. When talking about the badness of death, what we really mean should be the badness in sense (i). For the badness of death, according to deprivation theory, is completely *relational*[43], which is totally beyond our experiences or our attitudes. Therefore, it is more plausible for Brueckner and Fischer to maintain that the prenatal nonexistence is a bad thing. Particularly, since Brueckner and Fischer adopt objectivism—*value does not come from an individual's actually caring about something*—it would be very implausible for them to claim that prenatal nonexistence is not a bad thing.

To sum up, it is very problematic for Brueckner and Fischer to take the Posthumous harm approach.

In fact, there are at least two theoretical advantages for Brueckner and Fischer to take the Prenatal-and-Posthumous harm approach:

(1) They can explain the asymmetry in our *attitudes* toward prenatal and posthumous nonexistence.
(2) They can defend the deprivation view.

It seems that if Brueckner and Fischer take the Prenatal-and-Posthumous harm approach, they can therefore resolve the puzzles raised by Lucretius. Unfortunately, not only is this approach contrary to received wisdom, but also it is incorrect. For prenatal nonexistence is not a harm. This will be shown below.

III. Posthumous Harm Approach

Frances Myrna Kamm suggests a version of asymmetry to the effect that death is *worse* than prenatal nonexistence. She claims that there are three factors that explain why death is a harm: (i) the 'Injury factor' (or the 'Deprivation factor'), (ii) the 'Insult factor', and (iii) the 'Terror factor'. On the other hand, there is only one factor which accounts for the harm of prenatal nonexistence—the Injury factor. In other words, according to Kamm, the Insult factor and the Terror factor (neither of which is shared with prenatal nonexistence) explain why death is *worse* than prenatal nonexistence.[44] Let us examine these three factors now.

The Injury factor is described by Kamm as holding that '[death] eliminates further goods of life for the person who dies, goods that he would have had if he had lived.'[45]

She describes the Insult factor in these words:

> The Insult factor arises because death involves a loss of goods happening to a person who already exists. *Pre-natal non-existence deprives us of goods*, but not by, so to speak, confronting us when we already exist and undoing what we already are. In confronting us when we already exist and undoing what we already are, death but not prenatal non-existence takes away what we think of as already ours and also emphasizes our vulnerability.[46] (My emphasis.)

As to the Terror factor, Kamm describes this as follows:

> The Terror factor is connected with the fact that death is a permanent end to all significant periods of the person's life; there is no more possibility of such significant periods of life. This means that there is

no more possibility of goods of life for the person, but also simply no more possibility of the person himself existing (even without goods or with evils).[47]

I think that Kamm's proposal is problematic. Suppose these three factors are really factors for explaining the badness of death.[48] According to Kamm, the Injury factor can still apply to prenatal nonexistence. That is, Kamm, in fact, asserts that prenatal nonexistence is still a bad thing. With regard to this, Kamm says, 'The Deprivation Factor [i.e. the Injury factor]—independent of temporal location—does make both death and *prenatal nonexistence bad...*' [49] (My emphasis.)

However, as I will show below, the difference in value between death and prenatal nonexistence is not a matter of degree. By contrast, I will argue that prenatal nonexistence is not a harm. Therefore, Kamm's proposal cannot be accepted either.

Strictly speaking, Kamm's proposal is not a pure Posthumous harm approach. It is, in fact, a position in between the Posthumous harm approach and the Prenatal-and-Posthumous harm approach. Nagel's proposal, on the other hand, is purely a Posthumous harm approach.

Nagel argues that death is a harm whereas prenatal nonexistence is not. His reason is as follows:

> It is true that both the time before a man's birth and the time after his death are times when he does not exist. But the time after his death is time of which his death deprives him. It is time in which, had he not died then, he would be alive. Therefore any death entails the loss of *some* life that its victim would have led had he not died at that or any earlier point...
>
> But we cannot say that the time prior to a man's birth is time in which he would have lived had he been born not then but earlier. For aside from the brief margin permitted by premature labour, he *could not* have been born earlier: *anyone born substantially earlier than he was would have been someone else.* Therefore the time prior to his birth is not time in which his subsequent birth prevents him from living. His birth, when it occurs, does not entail the loss to him of any life whatever.[50] (My emphasis.)

Put simply, Nagel's point is that:

A person cannot be born earlier than he was—*because anyone born earlier would be someone else*—but a person could die later than he did. Therefore, the time prior to birth is not time of which that man has been deprived, whereas the time after death is.

If successful, Nagel's proposal would refute the 'symmetry thesis' (in the standard interpretation of the Lucretian symmetry argument) which has been widely criticised. In addition, this proposal, if sound, can explain the asymmetry in our attitudes toward death (i.e. posthumous nonexistence) and prenatal nonexistence: Since death is a harm, we look forward to it with dismay; while prenatal nonexistence is not a harm, so we are indifferent to it. However, Nagel's proposal has been widely criticised. The criticism tends to focus on his assertion that *a person born earlier than in fact he was would be a different person.*

Rosenbaum, for example, provides this blunt and clear attack:

> If the time at which we are born is essential to who we are, to our identity, why is not the time at which we die? If we could not have been born earlier (because if 'we' had been, 'we' would have been someone else), then we could not have died later (and still have been us).[51]

Nagel might respond as follows:

> According to the Kripkean view, a person's genetic origin is essential to the person's identity. That is, a person in fact originates with certain genetic material. Thus, if anyone born substantially earlier than he was, 'he' would have different genetic origin (i.e. he would be a different person).[52]

Rosenbaum criticises this supposed answer as follows:

(1) The Kripkean view that a person's genetic origin is essential to the person's personal identity is questionable.
(2) Suppose we grant the controversial view that a person's genetic origin is essential to the person's identity. Then, a particular sperm (with a specific genetic code) and a particular egg (with a specific genetic code) would be essential for a particular person, who comes into existence at specific time.

(3) On this supposition, for it to be *logically impossible* for the person to come into existence earlier, it would have to be *logically impossible* for the particular sperm and egg to exist at some earlier time and to fuse at some earlier time.

(4) However, this is *not logically impossible.*

(5) Therefore, it is *logically possible* that a person comes into being at some earlier time.[53]

I think the real issue here is over premise (4) in Rosenbaum's above argument—whether or not it is *logically impossible* for the particular sperm and egg to exist at some earlier time and to fuse at some earlier time. Most recent philosophers believe that it is *logically possible* for them to exist at some earlier time and to fuse at some earlier time. In short, they believe that a person can be born earlier. Brueckner and Fischer, for example, stress this position clearly:

> It is not clear that it is *logically impossible* that an individual should have been born substantially earlier than he actually was. It is not at all clear, for instance, that Socrates—the very same Socrates—could not (*logically*) have come into being ten years earlier than he in fact did.[54] (My emphasis.)

I think when or where one dies is a contingent fact. Similarly, when or where one exists along with what one does with his life is also a contingent fact. It might be physically impossible for a person to be born earlier. However, it is *logically* (or conceptually) possible for a person to be born earlier. Given this, it is reasonable for these recent philosophers to claim that the contingent fact—one's birth (or conception)—can (logically speaking) happen earlier. If they are correct in this point, then Nagel's proposal (i.e. the 'metaphysical personal identity approach') cannot be accepted.[55]

In the face of the above problems which Nagel confronts, Kaufman therefore modifies Nagel's metaphysical personal identity approach and adopts another approach—the 'psychological personal identity approach'. Kaufman believes that his new proposal (i.e. the psychological personal identity approach) can reject the symmetry thesis in the standard interpretation of the Lucretian symmetry argument (and, thus, the Lucretian symmetry argument). Let us now examine his proposal.

Kaufman suggests that 'person' can refer to: (1) member of the species *Homo sapiens* (a biological entity), or (2) an ongoing centre of self-awareness (a psychological entity). He emphasises that, in the discussions of death, the psychological features of persons are of greatest interest, rather than the biological.[56] In fact, contrary to Nagel, Kaufman concedes that it is possible for a person to have existed earlier, since genetic material could have occurred earlier. However, he argues that although a birth or a fertilisation or a bodily constitution could have occurred earlier, it does not show that, in the relevant sense, the same person could have existed earlier.[57] In other words, Kaufman maintains that it is the psychological personal identity, not the metaphysical personal identity, which is to the point in the discussions of death. To illustrate this, Kaufman writes:

> ...we see ourselves as persisting self-aware entities united by a continuity of memory. It is in virtue of psychological connectedness to the events of our lives that we construct a sense of ourselves as ourselves, and psychological continuity [i.e. the psychological personal identity] is what most concerns us when we deliberate about whether or not we could have lived at different times or different places; and the prospect of psychological extinction is surely what disturbs us when we think about death...
>
> An account of metaphysical personal identity in terms of origins, bodily continuity, and the like, does not require psychological continuity [i.e. the psychological personal identity]. But the relevant feature of personhood in the present context is psychological continuity [i.e. the psychological personal identity]...Since apparently it is possible to have metaphysical personal identity without psychological continuity [i.e. the psychological personal identity], and since *it is psychological continuity [i.e. the psychological personal identity] that concerns us in discussions of death*, there is no reason to think that an account of personal identity in terms of biological origins is relevant to the present inquiry.[58] (My emphasis.)

On the basis of this view, he suggests:

> To be told that a certain (biological) individual living 300 years from now will be me, in virtue of some genetic constitution or bodily continuity with my body now, is of little interest apart from my psychological continuity [i.e. the psychological personal identity]. Without my memories, psychology, and biography, a spatio-

temporal descendent of my body would remain *a complete stranger* to me.[59] (My emphasis.)

To sum up, Kaufman believes that in the discussions of death, the 'psychological personal identity' is of greatest interest.[60] Given this, here is the question: Is it possible for a person to exist earlier than in fact he did in terms of the psychological personal identity? To this question, Kaufman answers, 'No!' His reason for this answer is as follows:

> ...it is not possible for a person *in the psychological sense* to exist earlier than in fact he or she did because a psychological continuum [i.e. a psychological self] which, by hypothesis, starts earlier, would be a sufficiently different set of memories and experiences, and hence be a different psychological self. The contents of the biography of a person who exists in 1895 will be radically different from the biography of a person who exists in 1995; therefore, they cannot be the same (psychological) person, even if the genetic or bodily structure that exists in 1995 could have existed in 1895.[61] (My emphasis.)

He continues to say:

> Consider...what it would be like for *you* to have existed in 1895. You would recall, say, meeting Civil War veterans, encountering horseless carriages for the first time, and so forth. It is obvious that the contents of the psychological continuum [i.e. the psychological self] that would constitute the person whom your body would manifest if your body were around in 1895 would be completely different from the contents of the psychological continuum [i.e. the psychological self] you currently are. The person who would exist earlier would be *a complete stranger* to you.[62] (My emphasis.)

In short, Kaufman contends that imaginatively moving a person back in time would *disrupt* the psychological self with which we are *concerned*. However, he emphasises that there is no problem with imaginatively projecting the life of a person forward: to do so, we simply make additions to it. On the latter point, Kaufman says:

...extension of a self beyond the actual time of death is straightforward. Possible additions to the biography of a person who died in 1992 can be vividly imagined; perhaps the person visits Europe, perhaps the person marries and has children, and so forth. This is just the unfolding of the same life; and we can picture innumerable ways in which it might happen, but they all involve the same psychological person because we are making possible additions to a sequence that, up until the time of death, is already established. The psychological connectedness that that person has to his or her past is unaffected by the additional experiences.[63]

According to all this analysis, Kaufman concludes that a person cannot exist earlier than in fact he did, whereas a person could exist longer than he in fact does.[64]

If this conclusion is correct, then apparently the symmetry thesis in the standard interpretation of the Lucretian symmetry argument (and, thus, the Lucretian symmetry argument) should be rejected. Indeed, it seems that Kaufman's proposal is the most reasonable one among these proposals discussed so far. However, if we examine this proposal very carefully, we can still find some problems with it. The difficulty with Kaufman's proposal can be illustrated as follows.

Kaufman argues that we are not concerned about prenatal nonexistence, because we do not have any *psychological connectedness* to it.[65] Basically, this point is acceptable. However, it would be very contentious for him to conclude, from this point, that prenatal nonexistence is not a harm. Let me explain.

Indeed, I will be, as Kaufman describes, (nearly) indifferent to a mere spatio-temporal replica of my body 300 years in the future (if my counterpart will be in that possible world). On the other hand, my counterpart in that possible world would be (nearly) indifferent to me now in this actual world as well. By the same token, if *I* was born 20 years earlier than I actually was and raised in remote Alaska, then this Eskimo counterpart person, who spoke Aleut and lived in igloos, would be alien to me now. But note again that the Eskimo counterpart person in that possible world would also be indifferent to me now. And what this shows is *merely* that it is reasonable for us to have an indifferent attitude toward possible worlds to which we do not have any psychological connectedness. It would be very contentious to conclude, from this, that the possible world in which my counterpart will live 300 years later *is* not any good for 'me'—this counterpart person living 300 years later; or that the possible world in which my counterpart grew up in remote Alaska *is* not any good for 'me'—this Eskimo counterpart person. In contrast, it might be that certain possible worlds are better ones, and thus, I would rather choose them (if I could choose). To illustrate it, let us consider the following scenario originally from Nozick:

> Case One. Suppose people are all developed from individual spores that had existed indefinitely far in advance of their birth. In this fantasy, birth never occurs naturally more than a hundred years before the permanent end of the spore's existence. Now, we have discovered a way to trigger the premature hatching of these spores, and it is therefore possible for *me* to have been born 100 years earlier.[66]

In Case One, given that my actual life (like most other people's) is not extremely satisfactory for me now, I would be inclined to choose (if I could choose) the world in which I was born 100 years earlier. For I can therefore gain 100 years of life. To simplify discussion, I will assume that the goods of life are distributed evenly through time. That is, I assume that the longer life extends, the better life is for one. Consider another less fantastic example.

> Case Two. I was born in 1970 (I am now 30) and suppose I will naturally die in 2040. Suppose I could have been born 20 years earlier (i.e. in 1950) and die also in 2040. Suppose also that, in that possible world, it *is* 'now' 1980 and 'I' *am* 'now' 30. That is, 'I' *have* still 60 years to live.

In Case Two, I would choose (if I could choose) the (nonactual) possible world. It is true that I am (nearly) indifferent to that possible world. In a sense, I *do* lose my psychological self in that possible world. There is no psychological connectedness between me and 'me' (i.e. my counterpart in that possible world). However, in that possible world, 'I' also *gain* (in a sense) another identity (or psychological self). The fact that I do not care about that possible world should not be a reason for judging that that possible world is not any good for 'me' (i.e. my counterpart in that possible world). In just the same way 'I' (in that possible world) *do not care* about this actual world, but that should not be a reason for thinking that this is not a good world for me now.

Perhaps, one of the reasons against my above point is: Attempting imaginatively to picture *one's* coming into existence even several years earlier than one in fact did require one to think that he will be removed straightaway from this actual world to another world. That is, we might think that that new world would be very unfamiliar, uncertain, or even very unfriendly for him. In short, one would lose some psychological self in virtue of getting into a new world—e.g. losing a favourite friend, loved toys, or some very much cherished object.

In fact, Kaufman also endorses this view by saying:

> In short, imaginatively moving a person 'back' *disrupts* the psychological self...we must think that 'I want to live to see the middle of the 21st century' is coherent in a way that 'I want to have lived in the middle of the 19th century' is not. My desire to see the middle of the next century is perfectly sensible (even if unlikely) because I can clearly picture what it would be like for *me* to live to 2050. Nothing in my life up to this point will be any different and the imaginative projection of myself into the middle of the next century does *not disrupt* my biography...the projection involves additions to the continuum, not its *disruption*. But what would it be like for *me* to have lived in 1850? I would recall not only growing up in the last half of the twentieth century—my friends and family, the new playground at my element school, favourite television shows, etc.— but I would also remember the long journey to California in covered wagons across the prairie, shooting buffaloes and worrying about Indian attacks. *A coherent story of my inner life can scarcely be told.* This is because attempting imaginatively to project myself backward *disrupts* the sequence of experiences and memories to which I am currently psychologically connected.[67] (My emphasis.)

However, it should be emphasised here that this notion delivers an inappropriate picture in investigating the evaluation of the value of prenatal possible worlds. For the purpose of discussion, let me put another case which is revised from Case Two.

> Case Three. I was born in 1970 (I am now 30). Suppose I could have been born 20 years earlier (i.e. in 1950). Suppose also that, in that possible world, it *is* 'now' 1980 and 'I' *am* 'now' 30.

Indeed, as Kaufman asserts, in that prenatal possible world, 'I' would have (or be) another psychological self. 'I' might *gain* a lot of my biography from that possible world—e.g. encountering different friends, raising some loved pets, and so on. However, it is not appropriate to claim, from this, that imaginatively moving a person 'back' *disrupts* the psychological self. In contrast, it would be more appropriate to say that imaginatively moving a person 'back' generates another new and distinct psychological self. In short, in that possible world, there can definitely be some value in 'my' life—i.e. in the life of my counterpart in that possible world.

At this point, it is very important to note that once entertaining that possible world in which I was born earlier, we need to imagine that *this actual world would therefore no longer exist* (i.e. I no longer exist in the actual world). For it is implausible that a given individual may *actually* exist in both of these two worlds. In other words, it is inappropriate to imagine: Not only *do* I exist in this actual world, but I had also already lived in another possible world; and the value of that possible world is judged by me now (i.e. in 2000).

I suggest that we should evaluate the value of that possible world from the perspective of 'me' 'now' (i.e. in 1980) in that possible world, but not from the perspective of me now (i.e. in 2000) in this actual world. This just like we need to evaluate the actual world from my perspective now (i.e. in 2000) in this actual world, but not from 'my' perspective 'now' (i.e. in 1980) in that possible world. After all, it is 'I' who *live* in that possible world, but not I now (i.e. in 2000) who go into that possible world. According to this analysis, I would suggest further: *If that possible world has more goods for 'me' 'now' (i.e. in 1980) than the actual world has for me now (i.e. in 2000), then this prenatal nonexistence would be a harm to me. That is to say, it is a harm, in this case, for me not to be born 20 years earlier.*

Unfortunately, by sticking to the psychological personal identity approach, Kaufman completely ignores this point which is, I think, the key factor in evaluating the value of prenatal nonexistence.

Kaufman claims that it is not metaphysical personal identity which concerns us in the discussions of the evaluation of prenatal nonexistence. According to my above analysis, I would suggest that *it is not psychological personal identity either*. In contrast, I think, it is the comparison of the value of that prenatal possible world from the point view of my counterpart (in 1980) and the value of this real world from the point view of me now (in 2000) which concerns us in the discussions of the evaluation of prenatal nonexistence.

Accordingly, Kaufman's psychological personal identity approach cannot be accepted either. If so, then we need to find another way to reject the symmetry thesis in the standard interpretation of the Lucretian symmetry argument (and, thus, the Lucretian asymmetry argument).

I think that prenatal nonexistence is not a harm. Put simply, the reason for this is: *Prenatal nonexistence includes no facts with relation to the subject's interests.* Let me explicate this.

In fact, we simply do *not* expect to gain any more life in virtue of being born earlier, whereas we *do* know very well that we will gain some life due to the delay of our deaths. For more discussion, let us consider the following case:

> Case Four. Suppose 'I' was born in 1850. Suppose also that, in that possible world, it is 'now' 1880. 'I' *am* 'now' 30.

In that possible world, 'I' might, as Kaufman describes, experience the long journey to California in covered wagons across the prairie, shooting buffaloes and worrying about Indian attacks.[68] However, it is (biologically) impossible for 'me' to live until 2040. Yet, it would be, on the other hand, plausible for us to expect that 'I' would die in 1930 at the age of my 80. In short, although I might be eagerly willing to die later in order to live longer, I do not expect to live longer due to being born earlier. Conversely, in certain circumstances, I even think that it would be bad for me to be born earlier, such as in the following case:

> Consider the state of affairs of Mary being born in 1915. It is assumed that Mary's welfare level in that possible world *is* slightly lower than her welfare level in this actual world—after all, in that possible world she probably *endures* hard times during the Great Depression, and maybe even *catches* measles, whooping cough and other diseases that were rampant in those days. If she has just 50 years to live, it might be that she is better off living them in the second half of the twentieth century, rather than 35 years earlier.[69] (My emphasis.)

According to all this above analysis, it is concluded that *death is a harm in the way prenatal nonexistence is not.* Given this, it is plausible for us to be concerned about our death but indifferent to our prenatal nonexistence. For the delay of death would bring more life, whereas bringing birth forward would not.

In short, the symmetry thesis in the standard interpretation of the Lucretian symmetry argument (and, thus, the Lucretian asymmetry argument) is incorrect, and therefore should be rejected. If so, then the conclusion Chapter Four has reached—*death can be a harm to the person who dies*—would be unmoved.

5.3 FEAR OF DEATH

Cowards die many times before deaths;
The valiant never taste of death but once.
Of all the wonders that I yet have heard,
It seems to me most strange that man should fear;
Seeing that death, a necessary end,
Will come when it will come

--Shakespeare. *Julius Caesar*

Michael de Montaigne (1533-1592) writes, 'To philosophize is to learn to die.' [70] This remark forms part of a long-standing tradition in Western philosophy which teaches that a truly wise or rational man will not fear death. Such an idea is found in the Epicureans and the Stoics, among others. [71] Basically, their argument goes like this: Death is necessary or inevitable in the natural order of things and that, once one sees this, one will also see that it is irrational to fear death. [72] Baruch Spinoza (1632-1677) even emphasises that the absence of such irrational fearing is the mark of a kind of freedom or human liberation. He writes:

> A free man, that is to say, a man who lives according to the dictates of reason alone, is not led by fear of death, but directly desires the good, that is to say, desires to act, and to preserve his being in

accordance with the principle of seeking his own profit. He thinks, therefore, of nothing less than death, and his wisdom is a meditation upon life.[73]

On the other hand, given that death can be a harm as shown in Chapter Four, Section Two, it seems reasonable to claim that the fear of death is rational. Here, we face a puzzling and entangled issue.

To examine this issue, first of all it is very important to explicate the notion 'the fear of death'. The notion 'the fear of death' is crucially ambiguous.[74] There are at least two different meanings to the expression 'the fear of death': (1) the fear of necessary mortality and (2) the fear of premature death[75]. It is still under dispute whether the fear of necessary mortality is rational or not. On the other hand, the question, 'Is the fear of premature death rational?' has not been revolved settled yet.[76] To resolve these two questions, let us investigate a more basic question: 'When is a person rational in fearing?'

In his paper "Rationality and the Fear of Death", Jeffrie G. Murphy provides an account of the distinction between rational and irrational fearings as follows:

> It is rational for a person P to fear some state of affairs S if and only if:
> (1) P holds the reasonable belief that S obtains or is likely to obtain,
> (2) P holds the reasonable belief that S (a) is not easily avoided and (b) is very undesirable, bad, or evil for P,
> (3) the fear of S could be instrumental in bringing about some behavior or action that would allow P to avoid S, and
> (4) the fear of S is compatible, at least in the long run, with the satisfaction of the other important desires of P.[77]

With regard to condition (1), Murphy says:

> This, I take it, is the least controversial of the conditions I have put forth. Perhaps paradigm examples of people who suffer fears we regard as irrational are those who suffer from psychotic delusions. Paranoids, or alcoholics experiencing delirium tremens, for example, may fear the demons in the water faucets, the Martians in the closet, or the pink spiders on the wall. The best reason we have for thinking that these fears are irrational is the absence of any grounds or

evidence that there might be demons in the water faucets, Martians in the closet, or pink spiders on the wall.[78]

As to condition (2), Murphy writes:

> ...this condition also seems fairly noncontroversial...We should tend to characterize as irrational persons who are "scared to death" of (nonpoisonous) snakes or of high places. This is not because, as was the case in (1) above, there are no snakes or high places, but is rather because snakes and high places are normally harmless.[79]

Murphy illustrates condition (3) as follows:

> One way to characterize an activity as rational is to see that it has a point or purpose—that it at least appears to accomplish something. And surely it is avoidance behavior that gives fearing its significance...Fear's primary biological function is found in self-defensive behavior—what physiologists call the "fight or flight" reflex. And surely such fear, in addition to being biologically functional, is a part of what we understand by a rational approach to danger. If one discovers a hungry and aggressive tiger in the room, a state of affairs that surely satisfies conditions (1) and (2), who would doubt that the resulting fear is appropriate and that a person is rational in being "led" by the fear to the extent that he attempts to get out of the room as quickly as possible?[80]

As for (4), Murphy explicates:

> If the first three conditions are unsatisfied, we can perhaps, some may argue, conclude nothing more than that in such fearing the person is *non*rational. The present condition, however, surely gives us a test for genuine *ir*rationality with respect to fearing; and indeed its nonsatisfaction is a mark of fearings that we should call *neurotic*. A phobia, for example, becomes clearly a neurotic symptom, and not just something silly or eccentric, when it so pervades the life of the person who experiences it that he is rendered incapable of leading a successful and satisfying life.[81]

I think that Murphy's account of the distinction between rational and irrational fearings is acceptable. Given this account, the following conclusion would certainly be reached: the fear of *necessary* mortality is irrational. Let me explain.

First of all, many people believe that *immortality* is desirable or genuinely appealing to an individual. However, this view might be problematic. Williams, for example, asserts that death is not necessarily an evil. Indeed, according to Williams, it might even be that mortality is desirable in a sense.

Williams begins with a character in a play by Karel Capek which was made into an opera by Janacek. This character had various names with the initials 'EM'. When she was 42 years old, her father, the Court physician, gave her an elixir of life that rendered her capable of living forever (at the biological age of 42). At the time of action of the play, EM is aged 342. As Williams depicts, her unending life has come to a state of boredom, indifference, and coldness. Everything is joyless to her. In the end, she refuses to take the elixir again; she dies; and the formula is deliberately destroyed by a young woman (despite the protests of some older men).[82]

Here, Williams emphasises that there can be a worse state of affairs than death for an individual—a state of boredom. In other words, he believes that an endless life can be meaningless, i.e. immortality can be undesirable. Conversely, mortality might not be as bad as we perceive it to be. In a sense, death is required in order for life to be meaningful. Or, to put it in another way, death gives meaning to life. Without death, it seems that life would lack the structure in order for life to be meaningful. Thus, mortality might be desirable in so far as leading a meaningful life.

To reach the conclusion—the fear of necessary mortality is rational—each of the four conditions must be satisfied. However, if Williams' view is acceptable, then condition (2) might not well be satisfied although condition (1) is satisfied. Therefore, it might be problematic to claim that the fear of necessary mortality is rational.

Even if mortality is undesirable, condition (3) and perhaps condition (4) are unsatisfied.

Let us examine condition (3) first. It is assumed that we all die—no one can avoid mortality.[83] Given this assumption, clearly, the fear of our *necessary* mortality would definitely not result in our immortality. In short, our fear of *necessary* mortality is in vain.

As with condition (4), it is argued that the fear of necessary mortality can sometimes redound to our loss. For instance, to some people, the fear of necessary mortality can render them incapable of leading a normal and satisfying life. In this case, the fear of their own mortality is definitely not compatible, at least in the long run, with the satisfaction of their other important desires (e.g. to live a happy life).

According to the analyses above, the fear of necessary mortality is irrational.

Let us move on to the other issue over whether the fear of premature death is rational. On this issue, my answer is, 'Yes!' The reason for this assertive answer is explained as follows.

It is a fact that most people *do* die prematurely. How many people can be so lucky that they die at the limit of their natural biological life expectancy? It is also clear that the premature death is very undesirable, bad, or evil to us. Accordingly, both conditions (1) and (2) are satisfied

In addition, the fear of premature death could, at least indirectly, increase the probability of living close to the biological expectancy of life. In other words, the fear of premature death could serve as an instrument to greatly lessen the probability of our death during our prime. For example, the fear of premature death might lead one to maintain his health by exercising more and giving up smoking. Thus, condition (3) is also satisfied.

Besides, although the experience of the fear of premature death is an unpleasant one to have, it can be beneficial in a certain sense. Indeed, a prudential fear of premature death usually provokes people into maintaining a reasonable diligence with respect to living the kind of life they regard as proper or meaningful. In other words, it can aid us in avoiding bad things, such as interferences with the satisfactions that life offers.[84] In short, a prudential fear of our own mortality is compatible, at least in the long run, with the satisfaction of our other important desires (e.g. to live a happy life). If so, condition (4) is also satisfied.

The above analysis proves that the fear of premature death is rational. However, it should be emphasised that, in cases of neurotism, fears which are usually considered rational would become irrational. With respect to this, Murphy explicates:

> A certain fear of germs, for example, is certainly rational. There are germs, many germs are very harmful, and a fear of them can prompt a person to take reasonable precautions against disease. However, a person who is so afraid of germs that he washes twenty times a day, sprays all items in his house with germicide, refuses to leave his sanitized bedroom, etc., has crossed the boundary between reasonable prudence and irrational fearing.[85]

Therefore, although the fear of premature death is normally quite rational, it can become irrational when the fear becomes a neurotic one.

CONCLUSION

Although the Epicurean argument is a very powerful argument for resisting the common-sense view of death—generally a person's death is a great harm to him—I have shown, in Chapter One, that the Epicurean argument is defective. Hence, at this point, I can at least claim that it is possible that death *can* be a harm to the person who dies. However, to really secure this conclusion, it is necessary to give further justification.

There are two main theories which try to offer a direct reason for this conclusion: the desire-thwarting theory and the deprivation theory. In Chapter Two, I showed that the desire-thwarting theory is flawed. This suggests that the deprivation theory might be an acceptable theory to explain the badness of death.

In Chapter Three, I argued that, in general, if we singled out the cause of a person's death as causally closer to his death (i.e. to take a relatively narrower view of the cause of his death), then his death (event) would not be a harm and might even be a good thing for him. Conversely, if we singled out the cause of his death as causally further from his death (i.e. to take a relatively wider view of the cause of his death), then his death (event) would be a harm or even a tragedy for him.

In some circumstances, we are inclined to take a relatively narrower view of the cause of someone's death; while in other circumstances, we are inclined to take a relatively wider view. However, as I have shown in Chapter Three, we are inclined to, for the most part, take a relatively wider view of the cause of a person's death. Accordingly, it would be more accurate to state the conclusion of the deprivation theory as: 'death *as an event* is generally a harm to the person who dies from a relatively wider view of the cause of his death', rather than 'death is *generally* a harm to the person who dies', which is normally adopted by the deprivation theoriests.

In Chapter Three, I showed that, when considering the case of a person who dies prematurely, we can, and usually *do*, take two very different perspectives:

> (i) His death event (or the event which brings about his death) is a harm to him.
> (ii) His premature death (or the fact that he dies prematurely) is a harm to him.

As I have shown, a person's premature death (or the fact that a person dies prematurely) is *always* a harm to him. However, a person's death event (or the event which brings about a person's death) can be evaluated (on the deprivation theory) very differently depending on how we interpret this event (i.e. how we specify the cause of his death). According to the deprivation theory, the evaluation of a person's death event (or the event which brings about a person's death) can be: (1) a harm or even a tragedy for him, (2) a very *small* harm to him (i.e. hardly a harm to him), or even (3) a *good* thing for him. Accordingly, the evaluation of a person's premature death (or the fact that a person dies prematurely) can be quite inconsistent with the evaluation of his death event (or the event which brings about his death).

Although these two notions can be very different, they are, however, closely related. For example, in this case, his death event (no matter how we interpret it) will certainly bring about his premature death (or the fact that he dies prematurely). On the other hand, the notion of the death event and the notion of posthumous harms are also closely related. If we claim that P can be harmed by his own death event (or the event which brings about his own death), then we can also claim that he can be harmed by posthumous events. Indeed, these two claims are so related that we are obliged either to affirm both or to deny both.

Accordingly, in the case of a person who dies prematurely, the following three notions are actually strongly connected: the badness of his premature death (or the fact that he dies prematurely), the badness of his death event (or the event which brings about his death), and his posthumous harms. However, the deprivation theory can explain only the badness of his death event. Given this theoretical limitation, I therefore developed a more comprehensive theory (i.e. the interest-impairment theory) which could explain the following three closely related questions: (1) why a person's death event (or the event which brings about a person's death) is *generally* a harm to him from a relatively wider view of the cause of his death (or why a person's death event can be a harm to him), (2) why a person's premature death (or the fact that a person dies prematurely) is *always* a harm to him, and (3) why a person can be harmed posthumously.

To achieve this task, firstly, in Chapter Four, Section One, I briefly explicated the concept 'harm'. In that section, I showed that 'desire' is not suitable to explicate 'harm'. Given this, there is no surprise that the desire-thwarting theory should not be accepted. In contrast, 'harm' is best defined by the interest to the extent that *harm is the impairment of interest* (I called this the 'interest-impairment principle'). Unfortunately, in developing its account of the badness of death, the deprivation theory omits, or cannot account for, this essential characteristic of *harm*. This amounts to a serious limitation of the deprivation theory.

On the basis of the interest-impairment principle, I have justified in Chapter Four, Section Two the claim that a person's death event (or the event which brings about a person's death) from a relatively wider view of the cause of his death is *generally* a harm to him and the claim that a person's premature death (or the fact that a person dies prematurely) is *always* a harm to him. The reason for the claim that 'a person's death event (or the event which brings about a person's death) from a relatively wider view of the cause of his death is *generally* a harm to him' is as follows:

(i) Suppose P died at time T. It is certain that P's *death event* (or the event which brought about P's death) from a relatively wider view of the cause of his death directly blocked the continuation of his life (in the way he normally lived).

(ii) *In general*, the continuation of P's life (in the way he normally lived) was in his interests.

(iii) If (ii), then P's death event (or the event which brought about P's death) from a relatively wider view of the cause of his death, which blocked the continuation of his life (in the way he normally lived), would *certainly* have impaired P's interest.

(iv) *Harm is the impairment of interest.*

(v) Therefore, P's death event (or the event which brought about P's death) from a relatively wider view of the cause of his death, was *in general* a harm to him. Or at least, P's death event (or the event which brought about P's death) could be a harm to him.

On the other hand, the reason for the claim that a person's premature death (or the fact that a person dies prematurely) is *always* a harm to him is as follows:

(i) Suppose P died at his prime. His premature death (or the fact that he died prematurely) would entail the fact that he died before reaching his biological life expectancy.

(ii) To live a normally healthy life until our biological life expectancy is *always* in our interests.

(iii) Given (i) and (ii), P's premature death (or the fact that P died prematurely) would *always* impair his interest in living a normally healthy life until reaching his biological life expectancy.

(iv) *Harm is the impairment of interest.*

(v) Therefore, P's premature death (or the fact that P died prematurely) is *always* a harm to him.

In Chapter Four, Section Three, I continued to justify, by using the interest-impairment principle, the claim that a person could be harmed by posthumous events. To do this, firstly, I showed that some of a person's interests could survive the death of the person and thus could still be blocked. On the basis of this, secondly, I therefore reached the following conclusion that a person could be harmed by posthumous events. The reason for a person to be able to be harmed posthumously can be simply put as follows:

(i) A person's interests can survive the death of the person.

(ii) The interests which survive the death of a person may be impaired by posthumous events.

(iii) *Harm is the impairment of interest.*

(iv) Therefore, a person can be harmed by posthumous events.

These three arguments are essential components of the interest-impairment theory. By using the interest-impairment theory, I have thus reached the following three conclusions:

(1) A person's premature death (or the fact a person dies prematurely) is *always* a harm to him.

(2) A person's death event (or the event which brings about a person's death) from a relatively wider view on the cause of his death is *generally* a harm to him. Or at least, a person's death

event (or the event which brings about a person's death) can be a harm to him.

(3) A person can be harmed by *posthumous* events.

Given the conclusion (2), it is therefore concluded that death can be a harm to the person who dies.[1]

It seems that at this point I have fulfilled the purpose of this book. That is, I have justified the claim that death can be a harm to the person who dies. However, as I have emphasised in Introduction, to really justify this claim, it is necessary to further resolve two relevant puzzles raised especially by Epicureans:

(i) *Who* is the subject of the harm of death?

(ii) *When* is the subject harmed?

In Chapter Four, Section Three, I reached the conclusion that the subject of the harm of death is the *ante-mortem person*. In short, I have shown that there is no insoluble 'missing subject problem' as Epicureans insist.

If the subject of the harm of death is the *ante-mortem person*, then it implies that the subject has been harmed *before* death. Indeed, in Chapter Four, Section Four, I justified that it is really *before death* that the ante-mortem person is harmed by his own death.

Since I have shown the nature of the harm of death (by using the interest-impairment theory) and since I have also resolved these two puzzles, there is no problem for the claim that *death can be a harm to the person who dies.*

Following his master Epicurus, Lucretius addressed the task of proving that death is not a harm. Clearly, his conclusion directly challenges the conclusion I have already reached in Chapter Four—death can be a harm to the person who dies. The essential principle Lucretius adopts to reach his conclusion is the 'symmetry thesis'—both prenatal nonexistence and posthumous nonexistence (i.e. death) are not harms. There are a variety of recent philosophers who have tried to reject the symmetry thesis. Logically speaking, there are three possible approaches to rejecting the symmetry thesis:

(1) Showing that prenatal nonexistence is a harm, but death is not a harm.

(2) Showing that both prenatal nonexistence and death are harms.

(3) Showing that prenatal nonexistence is not a harm, but death is a harm.[2]

These three approaches can be called: (i) Prenatal harm approach, (ii) Prenatal-and-Posthumous harm approach, (iii) Posthumous harm approach.

In Chapter Five, Section Two, I first rejected the Prenatal harm approach and the Prenatal-and-Posthumous harm approach. Indeed, the Posthumous harm approach is the only correct approach. By taking the Prenatal-and-Posthumous harm approach, I refuted the symmetry thesis. The reason for the symmetry thesis to be flawed is: *Prenatal nonexistence includes no facts with relation to the subject's interests.* Or in more detail, since the delay of death would bring more life, death is a harm; whereas since bringing birth forward would not bring any life, prenatal nonexistence is not a harm.

Given that the Lucretian symmetry thesis, and thus, the Lucretian symmetry argument is incorrect, my position—death can be a harm to the person who dies—would be unmoved.

On the basis of the preceding discussion, I conclude that a person's death event (or the event which brings about a person's death) from a relatively wider view of the cause of his death is *generally* a harm to him. That is, *death can be a harm to the person who dies.*

Given this conclusion, it seems reasonable to claim that the fear of death is rational. However, this claim is challenged by a long-standing belief in western philosophy: Death is necessary or inevitable in the natural order of things and that, once one sees this, one will also see that it is irrational to fear death. To resolve this issue, first of all, I, in Chapter Six, Section Three, explicated the notion 'the fear of death'. After that, I argued: If 'death' is understood as premature death, then it is rational to fear it; whereas if 'death' is understood as necessary mortality, then it is irrational to fear it.

To sum up, there are three strong related questions about death:

(1) Is death a harm?
(2) Is premature death a harm?
(3) Can a posthumous event count as a harm?

My answers are:

(1) Death is *generally* a harm.
(2) Premature death is *always* a harm
(3) A posthumous event *can* count as a harm.

Because of the limitations of space, it is impossible to address all the related topics in such a book. Indeed, some of them deserve further extensive investigation. The following two topics are particularly important:

(1) The Appropriate Attitude towards Death: Given death is inevitable, how should we face or come to terms with it? If it is a harm or bad for us to fear death, then how can we philosophically or reflectively lessen or even transcend it?

(2) The Meaning of Death: Can death give meaning to life? That is, can death make life meaningful? If it can, then what kind of meaning can death bring to our lives? Is immortality desirable, insofar as leading a meaningful life is desirable?

In addition, there are further contentious moral issues pertaining to death which are worth exploring on the basis of the result of this book, in particular, moral problems relating to euthanasia or abortion.

With regard to euthanasia, we may at least ask: Should individuals, especially terminally ill people in excruciating pain (or the ones who are in an irreversibly coma), be able to end their lives? If no, why? If yes, may they hasten their deaths only by refuting medical treatment designed to sustain their lives, or may they take active measures to kill themselves? If they can take measures to kill themselves, can they ask others to assist them? Who can they ask: their spouses? close friends? their doctors? Should they expect the law to support their decisions?[3]

As to abortion, we may ask: Why would a woman have an abortion? What is the proper criterion of moral status? What is the moral status of the fetus? In other words, is the fetus a person? If it is, then the fetus has a serious right to life. Given the fetus has a serious right to life, is that sufficient to show that a woman must carry it to term? Must she do so even if she is seriously inconvenienced, or if her health is threatened? On the other hand, if the fetus is not a person (i.e. it is merely a human being), which is more important: (i) women's right to determine what happen in and to their bodies, or (ii) the fetus's right to life? Or up to what point of fetal development, if any, is abortion ethically acceptable?[4]

However, these are all tasks for another occasion.

NOTES

INTRODUCTION

1. Plato, *Phaedo*, 64a, trans. Hugh Tredennick, in *The Collected Dialogues of Plato*, eds. Edith Hamilton and Huntington Cairns (Princeton: Princeton University Press, 1961), p. 46.
2. This issue is too broad to be appropriately addressed with the scope of this book.
3. For a philosophical discussion of the possibility of an afterlife, see C. J. Ducasse, *A Critical Examination of the Belief in Life after Death* (Springfield: Illinois University Press, 1961); Terence Penelhum, *Survival and Disembodied Existence* (London: Routledge & K. Paul, 1970); Antony Flew, *Body, Mind, and Death* (New York: Macmillan, 1964); and John Hick, *Death and Eternal Life* (London: Collins, 1976).
4. See Joel Feinberg, 'Harm to Others', in *The Metaphysics of Death*, ed. John Martin Fischer (Stanford: Stanford University Press, 1993), p. 171; and Jeff McMahan, 'Death and the Value of Life', in *The Metaphysics of Death*, ed. John Martin Fischer (Stanford: Stanford University Press, 1993), pp. 233-234.
5. Throughout this book I use 'he', 'him', or 'his' as gender-neutral pronouns.
6. See 'Introduction: Death, Metaphysics, and Morality', in *The Metaphysics of Death*, ed. John Martin Fischer (Stanford: Stanford University Press, 1993), p. 4.
7. Ibid., p. 6. For discussions of the biological approach, see Lawrence C. Becker, 'Human Being: The Boundaries of the Concept', *Philosophy and Public Affairs* 4 (1975), pp. 335-359; and David Lamb, 'Diagnosing Death', *Philosophy and Public Affairs* 7 (1978), pp. 144-153.
8. 'Introduction: Death, Metaphysics, and Morality', in *The Metaphysics of Death*, ed. John Martin Fischer (Stanford: Stanford University Press, 1993), p. 6. For discussions of the moral approach, see Hans Jonas, *Philosophical Essays: From Ancient Creed to Technological Man* (Englewood Cliffs: Prentice-Hall, Inc., 1974); Howard Brody, *Ethical Decisions in Medicine*, 2nd ed. (Boston: Little, Brown and Company, 1981); and Howard Brody, 'Brain

Death and Personal Existence: A Reply to Green and Wikler', *Journal of Medicine and Philosophy* 8 (1983), pp. 187-196.

9. 'Introduction: Death, Metaphysics, and Morality', in *The Metaphysics of Death,* ed. John Martin Fischer (Stanford: Stanford University Press, 1993), pp. 6-7. For discussions of the metaphysical approach, see Michael B. Green and Daniel Wikler, 'Brain Death and Personal Identity', *Philosophy and Public Affairs* 9 (1980), pp. 105-133; George J. Agich and Royce P. Jones, 'Personal Identity and Brain Death: A Critical Response', *Philosophy and Public Affairs* 15 (1986), pp. 267-274; and Karen Grandstrand Gervais, *Redefining Death* (New Haven: Yale University Press, 1986).

10. For a discussion of this view, see L. W. Sumner, 'A Matter of Life and Death', *Nous* 10 (1976), pp. 154-157; and Jeff McMahan, 'Death and the Value of Life', in *The Metaphysics of Death,* ed. John Martin Fischer (Stanford: Stanford University Press, 1993), fn. 2.

11. See Stephen E. Rosenbaum, 'How to Be Dead and Not Care: A Defence of Epicurus', in *The Metaphysics of Death,* ed. John Martin Fischer (Stanford: Stanford University Press, 1993), p. 121.

12. Rosenbaum also makes a similar point. See Stephen E. Rosenbaum, 'The Harm of Killing: An Epicurean Perspective', in *Contemporary Essays on Greek Ideas: The Kilgore Festschrift,* eds. Robert M. Baird, William F. Cooper, Elmer H. Duncan, and Stuart E. Rosenbaum (Waco: Baylor University Press, 1987), pp. 208-209.

13. See L. W. Sumner, 'A Matter of Life and Death', *Nous* 10 (1976), pp. 153-154. For an interesting discussion of this topic, see Jeff McMahan, 'Death and the Value of Life', in *The Metaphysics of Death,* ed. John Martin Fischer (Stanford: Stanford University Press, 1993), pp. 259-261.

14. See 'The Makropulos Case: Reflections on the Tedium of Immortality', in Bernard Williams, *Problems of the Self* (Cambridge: Cambridge University Press, 1973), pp. 85-86; and Steven Luper-Foy, 'Annihilation', in *The Metaphysics of Death,* ed. John Martin Fischer (Stanford: Stanford University Press, 1993), pp. 270-276.

15. See Fred Feldman, 'Some Puzzles about the Evil of Death', in *The Metaphysics of Death,* ed. John Martin Fischer (Stanford: Stanford University Press, 1993), p. 308; Palle Yourgrau, 'The Dead', in *The Metaphysics of Death,* ed. John Martin Fischer (Stanford: Stanford University Press, 1993), p. 140; Anthony L. Brueckner and John Martin Fischer, 'Why Is Death Bad?', in *The Metaphysics of Death,* ed. John Martin Fischer (Stanford:

Stanford University Press, 1993), p. 222; and 'Death', in Thomas Nagel, *Mortal Questions* (London: Cambridge University Press, 1979).

16. By 'premature death', I mean the fact that people die before their natural biological life expectancy. According to this definition, if a person dies in his prime, he dies prematurely. On the other hand, if an old person dies at the limit of his natural biological life expectancy, he does not die prematurely. Unfortunately, however, most people *do* die prematurely. Note further that premature death as I mean here is different from the death event (or the event which brings about death) which happens while there is still the prospect of a worthwhile life for us.

17. See Joel Feinberg, 'Harm to Others', in *The Metaphysics of Death,* ed. John Martin Fischer (Stanford: Stanford University Press, 1993), p. 174.

18. See Lucretius, *On the Nature of Things,* trans H.A.J. Munro, in *The Stoic and Epicurean Philosophers,* ed. Whitney Jennings Oates (New York: Modern Library, 1957), p. 131.

19. See 'Death', in Thomas Nagel, *Mortal Questions* (London: Cambridge University Press, 1979), pp. 7-8.

20. See Frederik Kaufman, 'Death and Deprivation; or, Why Lucretius' Symmetry Argument Fails', *Australasian Journal of Philosophy* 74 (1996), pp. 305-312.

21. See Jeffrie G. Murphy, 'Rationality and the Fear of Death', in *The Metaphysics of Death,* ed. John Martin Fischer (Stanford: Stanford University Press, 1993), p. 44.

CHAPTER ONE

1. See Harry S. Silverstein, 'The Evil of Death', in *The Metaphysics of Death,* ed. John Martin Fischer (Stanford: Stanford University Press, 1993), p. 95.

2. For a discussion of Epicurus' philosophical background, see J. M. Rist, *Epicurus: An Introduction* (Cambridge: Cambridge University Press, 1972). See also P. H. De Lacy, 'Epicurus', in *Encyclopedia of Philosophy,* vol. 3, ed. Paul Edwards (New York: Macmillan, 1967).

3. Epicurus, 'Letter to Menoeceus', trans. C. Bailey, in *The Stoic and Epicurean Philosophers,* ed. Whitney Jennings Oates (New York: Modern Library, 1957), pp. 30-31. Epicurus, in this argument, apparently raises two reasons to support his conclusion—death is nothing to us: (1) When we are,

death is not come, and (2) When death is come, we are not. However, reason (1) is not strong enough to support Epicurus' conclusion, because the *expectation of death* may be a harm or misfortune for the living. Perhaps this is a rhetorically provocative and somewhat exaggerated way of expressing his basic idea about death. Anyhow, reason (1) is entirely irrelevant to the argument. Therefore, I will follow most philosophers, especially Rosenbaum, and ignore it.

4. See Jeff McMahan, 'Death and the Value of Life', in *The Metaphysics of Death,* ed. John Martin Fischer (Stanford: Stanford University Press, 1993), pp. 233-234; and Joel Feinberg, 'Harm to Others', in *The Metaphysics of Death,* ed. John Martin Fischer (Stanford: Stanford University Press, 1993), p. 171.

5. This reconstruction is based on Rosenbaum's text which I have slightly modified. In his reconstruction of the Epicurean argument, Rosenbaum presupposes that there is a tertiary stage intervening between dying and death (being dead). However, it is not clear whether such a stage exists. Even if it exists, the characteristics of this stage are still unclear. According to Rosenbaum, this stage is roughly the time at which a person becomes dead. However, it is not clear that it is a stage of a person's life. It is not clear that it takes time or, if so, how much time it takes. It may be a mere moment in time separating dying from death (being dead). Most importantly, it is not clear whether or not there is a subject left during this stage; nor is it clear, if there is a subject, what the characteristics of this subject are or in what sense it is a subject. Given this, to simplify our discussion, in my reconstruction of the Epicurean argument, I suppose that there are only two stages in one's history: dying and death (being dead). See Stephen E. Rosenbaum, 'How to Be Dead and Not Care: A Defence of Epicurus', in *The Metaphysics of Death,* ed. John Martin Fischer (Stanford: Stanford University Press, 1993), pp. 120-122.

6. Fischer, McMahan, Silverstein, and William Grey, for example, also (broadly speaking) accept this reconstruction. See 'Introduction: Death, Metaphysics, and Morality', in *The Metaphysics of Death,* ed. John Martin Fischer (Stanford: Stanford University Press, 1993), pp. 1-30; Jeff McMahan, 'Death and the Value of Life', in *The Metaphysics of Death,* ed. John Martin Fischer (Stanford: Stanford University Press, 1993), pp. 233-266; Harry S. Silverstein, 'The Evil of Death', in *The Metaphysics of Death,* ed. John Martin Fischer (Stanford: Stanford University Press, 1993), pp. 95-116; and William Grey, 'Epicurus and the Harm of Death', *Australasian Journal of Philosophy* 77 (1999), pp. 358-364.

7. Usually, there are difficulties in interpreting classic works. It might be found that there are inconsistent notions or even theories in a classic author's works. This is partly caused by the usage of vague language, missing parts of the author's works, loss in translation, or even the existence of spurious works. It might prove very difficult to have a completely precise understanding of what Epicurus really meant by this argument. However, the philosophical importance of these issues extends beyond the question of the historical accuracy of interpretations of the Epicurean argument and the philosophical insights which it contains. In the light of this, I accept Rosenbaum's reconstruction of the Epicurean argument as appropriate, even though he may misunderstand Epicurus' original intentions. I provide only a very slight revision of Rosenbaum's argument.

8. John Woods also draws a clear distinction between 'death' and 'dying'. He says:

> The fear of death is not the fear of dying, with which it is sometimes confused. To fear *dying* is to fear living through the usually rather trying concluding episodes of one's existence. To fear *death* is to fear the circumstance of one's nonexistence, not the experience of its approach. Fear of death is fear of the void...

John Woods, 'Can Death Be Understood', in *Values and the Quality of Life*, eds. William R. Shea and John King-Farlow (New York: Science History Publications, 1976), p. 161.

9. 'Introduction: Death, Metaphysics, and Morality' in *The Metaphysics of Death,* ed. John Martin Fischer (Stanford: Stanford University Press, 1993), p. 4.

10. Kaufman also makes this point. He says, 'It is clear that Epicurus is talking about being dead, not the process of dying, which can be awful and hence rationally feared.' Frederik Kaufman, 'Death and Deprivation; or, Why Lucretius' Symmetry Argument Fails', *Australasian Journal of Philosophy* 74 (1996), fn. 1.

11. See Stephen E. Rosenbaum, 'How to Be Dead and Not Care: A Defence of Epicurus', in *The Metaphysics of Death,* ed. John Martin Fischer (Stanford: Stanford University Press, 1993), p. 121; and 'Introduction: Death, Metaphysics, and Morality' in *The Metaphysics of Death,* ed. John Martin Fischer (Stanford: Stanford University Press, 1993), pp. 3-4.

12. Stephen E. Rosenbaum, 'How to Be Dead and Not Care: A Defense of Epicurus', in *The Metaphysics of Death,* ed. John Martin Fischer (Stanford: Stanford University Press, 1993), pp. 122-123.

13. Ibid., pp. 120-121.

14. Julian Lamont, 'A Solution to the Puzzle of When Death Harms Its Victims', *Australasian Journal of Philosophy* 76 (1998), p. 210.

15. Epicurus, 'Letter to Menoeceus', trans. C. Bailey, in *The Stoic and Epicurean Philosophers*, ed. Whitney Jennings Oates (New York: Modern Library, 1957), pp. 30-31.

16. See Stephen E. Rosenbaum, 'How to Be Dead and Not Care: A Defense of Epicurus', in *The Metaphysics of Death,* ed. John Martin Fischer (Stanford: Stanford University Press, 1993), p. 124.

17. Ibid.

18. Ibid.

19. Step (C) in the standard interpretation of the Epicurean argument can be found at the beginning of this section.

20. See Jeff McMahan, 'Death and the Value of Life', in *The Metaphysics of Death,* ed. John Martin Fischer (Stanford: Stanford University Press, 1993), pp. 233-234.

21. Ibid., p. 234.

22. Here, I suppose Epicurus would have chosen to make his view reasonable and consistent. It is for this reason that I assume that we need to specify a more precise necessary condition in the Epicurean argument.

23. See Harry S. Silverstein, 'The Evil of Death', in *The Metaphysics of Death,* ed. John Martin Fischer (Stanford: Stanford University Press, 1993), p. 96.

24. Epicurus, 'Letter to Menoeceus', trans. C. Bailey, in *The Stoic and Epicurean Philosophers*, ed. Whitney Jennings Oates (New York: Modern Library, 1957), p. 30.

25. When I claim that 'P can experience a state of affairs (or event)' is a more precise necessary condition than 'P exists when a state of affairs (or event) occurs', I do not mean that the latter is not a precise necessary condition for that state of affairs (or event) being a harm (or bad thing) for P. What I mean is that: the reason for 'P exists when a state of affairs (or event) occurs' to be a necessary condition for that state of affairs (or event) being a harm (or bad thing) for P is based on the supposition that 'P can experience a state of affairs (or event)' is a necessary condition for that state of affairs (or event) being a harm (or bad thing) for P. Put it another way, 'P can

experience a state of affairs (or event)' is a more precise statement of necessary condition for that state of affairs (or event) being a harm (or bad) for P.

26. Someone might argue that 'P exists when a state of affairs (or event) occurs' is a *necessary and sufficient* condition for 'P can experience the state of affairs (or event)', so it is claimed that 'P can experience a state of affairs (or event)' is not a more precise *necessary* condition for the state of affairs (or event) being a harm (or bad thing) for P than 'P exists when the state of affairs (or event) occurs'. To this challenge, I have the following response:

> (1) It is very difficult to judge whether, in the Epicurean argument, 'P exists when a state of affairs (or event) occurs' is a *necessary and sufficient* condition for 'P can experience the state of affairs (or event)'. However, it is clear that 'P exists when a state of affairs (or event) occurs' is a necessary condition for 'P can experience the state of affairs (or event)'. Thus, 'P does not exist when a state of affairs (or event) occurs' would exclude the possibility that 'P can experience the state of affairs (or event)'.
>
> (2) 'Experience' is conceptually more relevant to 'harm' or 'bad' than 'existence'.

Therefore, even if 'P exists when a state of affairs (or event) occurs' is a *necessary and sufficient* condition for 'P can experience the state of affairs (or event)', I can still claim that conceptually 'P can experience a state of affairs (or event)' is a more precise necessary condition for the state of affairs (or event) being a harm (or bad thing) for P than 'P exists when the state of affairs (or event) occurs'.

It is in this sense that I claim: 'P can experience a state of affairs (or event)' is a more precise necessary condition for the state of affairs (or event) being a harm (or bad thing) for P than 'P exists when the state of affairs (or event) occurs'.

27. Stephen E. Rosenbaum, 'How to Be Dead and Not Care: A Defence of Epicurus', in *The Metaphysics of Death,* ed. John Martin Fischer (Stanford: Stanford University Press, 1993), p. 123.

28. This weaker sense of 'possibility' in (3) is identified by Fischer which he calls the 'narrow' sense of possibility. See John Martin Fischer, 'Death, Badness, and the Impossibility of Experience', *Journal of Ethics* 1 (1997), p. 347.

29. P. H. De Lacy, in explicating the philosophy of Epicurus, writes, 'The feelings of pleasure and pain that accompany sense experiences are the ultimate good and evil; all statements about good and evil are meaningful only by reference to these feelings.' This can be seen to support the conclusion I reach about the Epicurean argument. See P. H. De Lacy, 'Epicurus', in *Encyclopedia of Philosophy*, vol. 3, ed. Paul Edwards, p. 3.

30. Maybe I should put (4) as: 'P experiences and feels a state of affairs (or event) as bad when the state of affairs (or event) occurs' is a *sufficient and necessary* condition for the state of affairs (or event) being a harm (or bad thing) for P; whereas 'P experiences and feels a state of affairs (or event) as good when the state of affairs (or event) occurs' is a *sufficient and necessary* condition for the state of affairs (or event) being a good thing for P. However, to refute the Epicurean argument, it is enough to put (4) as: 'P experiences and feels a state of affairs (or event) as bad when the state of affairs (or event) occurs' is a *sufficient* condition for the state of affairs (or event) being a harm (or bad thing) for P; whereas 'P experiences and feels a state of affairs (or event) as good when the state of affairs (or event) occurs' is a *sufficient* condition for the state of affairs (or event) being a good thing for P.

31. 'Death', in Thomas Nagel, *Mortal Questions* (London: Cambridge University Press, 1979), p. 3.

32. Cf. Steven Luper-Foy, 'Annihilation', in *The Metaphysics of Death*, ed. John Martin Fischer (Stanford: Stanford University Press, 1993), p. 274.

33. Cf. 'Death', in Thomas Nagel, *Mortal Questions* (London: Cambridge University Press, 1979), p. 4.

34. George Pitcher, 'The Misfortunes of the Dead', in *The Metaphysics of Death*, ed. John Martin Fischer (Stanford: Stanford University Press, 1993), p. 165.

35. Cf. Julian Lamont, 'A Solution to the Puzzle of When Death Harms Its Victims', *Australasian Journal of Philosophy* 76 (1998), p. 207.

36. Jeff McMahan, 'Death and the Value of Life', in *The Metaphysics of Death*, ed. John Martin Fischer (Stanford: Stanford University Press, 1993), p. 235.

37. Ibid., pp. 240-241.

38. The Epicurean argument is also discussed by David Hume (1711-1776). See James Boswell, 'An Account of My Last Interview with David Hume, Esq.', in *Private Papers of James Boswell* (Isham Collection), p. 229.

CHAPTER TWO

1. I know the notion of desire and the notion of wish are different in a strict sense. To simply our discussion, I, following most desire-thwarting theorists, use 'desire' to mean: desire, want, or wish.
2. See Steven Luper-Foy, 'Annihilation', in *The Metaphysics of Death,* ed. John Martin Fischer (Stanford: Stanford University Press, 1993), pp. 270-271.
3. 'The Makropulos Case: Reflections on the Tedium of Immortality', in Bernard Williams, *Problems of the Self* (Cambridge: Cambridge University Press, 1973), p. 85.
4. See Ibid., pp. 85-86.
5. See Steven Luper-Foy, 'Annihilation', in *The Metaphysics of Death,* ed. John Martin Fischer (Stanford: Stanford University Press, 1993), p. 276.
6. 'The Makropulos Case: Reflections on the Tedium of Immortality', in Bernard Williams, *Problems of the Self* (Cambridge: Cambridge University Press, 1973), p. 85.
7. 'Introduction: Death, Metaphysics, and Morality', in *The Metaphysics of Death,* ed. John Martin Fischer (Stanford: Stanford University Press, 1993), p. 16.
8. See Steven Luper-Foy, 'Annihilation', in *The Metaphysics of Death,* ed. John Martin Fischer (Stanford: Stanford University Press, 1993), p. 276.
9. See 'The Makropulos Case: Reflections on the Tedium of Immortality', in Bernard Williams, *Problems of the Self* (Cambridge: Cambridge University Press, 1973), p. 87. Ruth Cigman also sheds a light on this point by comparing 'the death of a person' (which is a misfortune) with 'the death of an animal' (which, she argues, is not a misfortune because animals cannot have categorical desires). See Ruth Cigman, 'Death, Misfortune and Species Inequality', *Philosophy and Public Affairs* 10 (1981), pp. 47-64.
10. Steven Luper-Foy, 'Annihilation', in *The Metaphysics of Death,* ed. John Martin Fischer (Stanford: Stanford University Press, 1993), p. 275.
11. Ibid.
12. 'Introduction: Death, Metaphysics, and Morality', in *The Metaphysics of Death,* ed. John Martin Fischer (Stanford: Stanford University Press, 1993), p. 17.
13. In some very special circumstances, it is possible for someone to have no unconditional desires, and, thus, (2) might be challenged. However, for most healthy people, in most circumstances, the death (event) *does* thwart

certain kind(s) of their *unconditional* desires. Thus, (2) can be generally accepted. In short, (2) is not the essential problem in the desire-thwarting argument. To respond to this challenge, we at most need to have a slight modification for the desire-thwarting argument as follows:

(i) Something is a harm or misfortune for us if it thwarts any of our desires.

(ii) Death is a harm or misfortune for us, *if* it thwarts certain kind(s) of our unconditional desires.

Even (2) is understood in this way, I would say that the desire-thwarting theory is still seriously flawed. See 'Introduction: Death, Metaphysics, and Morality', in *The Metaphysics of Death*, ed. John Martin Fischer (Stanford: Stanford University Press, 1993), p.18.

14.   See Joel Feinberg, 'Harm to Others', in *The Metaphysics of Death*, ed. John Martin Fischer (Stanford: Stanford University Press, 1993), p.177. The distinction between fulfilment and satisfaction was made originally by W. D. Ross, *Foundations of Ethics* (Oxford: Clarendon, 1939), p. 300.

15.   Joel Feinberg, 'Harm to Others', in *The Metaphysics of Death*, ed. John Martin Fischer (Stanford: Stanford University Press, 1993), p.177.

16.   Ibid.

17.   Ibid., p. 178.

18.   See Ibid.

19.   See Ibid.

20.   Derek Parfit, *Reasons and Persons*, relevant passage in *The Metaphysics of Death*, ed. John Martin Fischer (Stanford: Stanford University Press, 1993), p. 202.

21.   Stephen E. Rosenbaum, 'Epicurus and Annihilation', in *The Metaphysics of Death*, ed. John Martin Fischer (Stanford: Stanford University Press, 1993), p.300.

22.   See Ibid.

CHAPTER THREE

1. See Fred Feldman, 'Some Puzzles about the Evil of Death', in *The Metaphysics of Death*, ed. John Martin Fischer (Stanford: Stanford University Press, 1993), p. 308.

2. See Harry S. Silverstein, 'The Evil of Death', in *The Metaphysics of Death*, ed. John Martin Fischer (Stanford: Stanford University Press, 1993), p. 98.

3. 'Death', in Thomas Nagel, *Mortal Questions* (London: Cambridge University Press, 1979), p. 1.

4. Ibid., pp. 3-4.

5. 'The Makropulos Case: Reflections on the Tedium of Immortality', in Bernard Williams, *Problems of the Self* (Cambridge: Cambridge University Press, 1973), p. 84.

6. L. W. Sumner, 'A Matter of Life and Death', *Nous* 10 (1976), pp. 157-158.

7. See Fred Feldman, 'Some Puzzles about the Evil of Death', in *The Metaphysics of Death,* ed. John Martin Fischer (Stanford: Stanford University Press, 1993), p. 308. This account is also accepted by Palle Yourgrau. He says:

> Death, clearly, will be an evil...But what is it the dead relate to, which explains their misfortune? Surely it is precisely the life they have been denied—the possibility of enjoying all that life is a precondition for.

Palle Yourgrau, 'The Dead', in *The Metaphysics of Death,* ed. John Martin Fischer (Stanford: Stanford University Press, 1993), p. 140. Anthony L. Brueckner and John Martin Fischer also argue for the same point as follows:

> Death could then be an *experiential blank* and still be a bad thing for an individual...why this is so is that death (although an experiential blank) is *deprivation* of the good things of life. That is, when life is, on balance, good, then death is bad insofar as it robs one of this good: if one had died later than one actually did, then one would have had more of the good things of life.

Anthony L. Brueckner and John Martin Fischer, 'Why Is Death Bad?', in *The Metaphysics of Death,* ed. John Martin Fischer (Stanford: Stanford University Press, 1993), p. 222. Similar views are defended or at least discussed by a number of philosophers. See, for example, 'Death', in Thomas Nagel, *Mortal Questions* (London: Cambridge University Press, 1979); Jeff McMahan, 'Death and the Value of Life', in *The Metaphysics of Death,* ed. John Martin Fischer (Stanford: Stanford University Press, 1993); L. W. Sumner, 'A Matter of Life and Death', *Nous* 10 (1976), pp. 145-171; 'The Makropulos Case: Reflections on the Tedium of Immortality', in Bernard Williams, *Problems of the Self* (Cambridge: Cambridge University Press, 1973); Douglas N. Walton, *On Defining Death: An Analytic Study of the Concept of Death in Philosophy and Medical Ethics* (Montreal: McGill-Queen's University Press, 1979); and Roy W. Perrett, *Death and Immortality* (Boston: Martinus Nijhoff Publishers, 1987).

8. Apparently, the deprivation theory has assumed that life, in general, is good. This assumption can also be found in McMahan's illustration of the deprivation theory. McMahan says:

> Death is bad for a person…Other things being equal, the badness of death is proportional to…the goods of [life] of which the victim is deprived.

Jeff McMahan, 'Death and the Value of Life', in *The Metaphysics of Death,* ed. John Martin Fischer (Stanford: Stanford University Press, 1993), p. 262. Because of this, Sumner contends:

> To answer fully the question why death is generally an evil we must therefore determine why life is generally a good.

L. W. Sumner, 'A Matter of Life and Death', *Nous* 10 (1976), p. 158.

Accordingly, to justify 'the general good of life' is therefore to further justify the deprivation theory. Indeed, some deprivation theorists, such as Nagel and Sumner, have tried to prove this assumption. However, I do not believe that they have fully and successfully *justified* this assumption. It is not even clear that this assumption *can* be justified. Anyhow, this issue is too large to be taken up here: it would be too daunting a task for me to attempt to provide an adequate analysis of this issue within the confines of this book. I will therefore just presuppose this assumption in my discussion of the deprivation theory.

To examine the deprivation theorists' arguments for this assumption, see L. W. Sumner, 'A Matter of Life and Death', *Nous* 10 (1976), pp. 158-160; and 'Death', in Thomas Nagel, *Mortal Questions* (London: Cambridge University Press, 1979), pp. 1-2.

9. See 'Death', in Thomas Nagel, *Mortal Questions* (London: Cambridge University Press, 1979), p.1.

10. Ibid., pp. 4-5.
11. Robert Nozick, 'On the Randian Argument', in *Reading Nozick: Essays on Anarchy, State, and Utopia*, ed. Jeffrey Paul (Oxford: Blackwell, 1982), p. 221.
12. See 'Introduction: Death, Metaphysics, and Morality', in *The Metaphysics of Death*, ed. John Martin Fischer (Stanford: Stanford University Press, 1993), pp. 20-21.
13. See Ibid., pp. 21-22; and Frederik Kaufman, 'Pre-Vital and Post-Mortem Non-Existence', *American Philosophical Quarterly* 36 (1999), pp. 2-4.

In his recent paper 'Death, Badness, and the Impossibility of Experience', Fischer distinguishes two principles which are generally used by the critics of the deprivation theory (of course, including Epicureans) to refute the deprivation theory:

> (1) Experience Requirement I (ER I): An individual can be harmed by something only if he has an unpleasant experience as a result of it (either directly or indirectly).
> (2) Experience Requirement II (ER II): An individual can be harmed by something only if it is possible for him to have an unpleasant experience as a result of it (either directly or indirectly).

In support of his position (i.e. the deprivation theory), Nagel raises his betrayal example. However, suggests Fischer, Nagel's betrayal example can impugn only ER I, and not ER II. Further, these critics have emphasised that ER II appears to imply that death is not a harm to the person who dies. Thus, it is alleged that Nagel's betrayal example (and, of course, all those examples in the above two arguments) fall short of establishing that death can be a harm to an individual. In the face of this, Fischer therefore tries to raise a counterexample to ER II to defend the deprivation theory. That is, he tries to suggest a non-question-begging example in which an individual *cannot* have an unpleasant experience as a result of something and yet we would say that that thing is a harm or bad for the individual. Fischer puts his example as follows:

> Imagine first that the example is as described by Nagel. You are betrayed behind your back by people who you thought were good friends, and you never actually find out about this or have any bad

experiences as a result of the betrayal. But now suppose that these friends were (very) worried that you might find out about the betrayal. In order to guard against this possibility, they arrange for White to watch over you. His task is to prevent you ever from finding out about the betrayal. So, for example, if one of the individuals who betrayed you should decide to tell you about it, White can prevent him from succeeding: White can do whatever is required to prevent the information from getting to you. Or if you should begin to seek out one of the friends, White could prevent you from succeeding in making contact. I simply stipulate that White is in a position to thwart any attempt by you or your friends to inform you of what happened.

In this Frankfurt-style version of Nagel's betrayal example, I further stipulate that everything (plausibly thought to be relevant) that actually happens among your friends and to you (and your family) is exactly the same as in the original version of the example; we could 'subtract' the existence of White and this would make *no relevant difference* to what actually happens among your friends and to you (and your family) for the rest of your life. The *only* difference between the original case and the modified case is that your friends have so arranged things that White is poised to intervene at any point in your life where there would be a chance that you would discover what happened; it turns out that intervention is never actually necessary, and thus the actual sequence of events in the modified example is in relevant respects precisely like that of the original example. White serves as a fail-safe mechanism; his intervention is never triggered, but his presence ensures that you will never find out about the betrayal.

John Martin Fischer, 'Death, Badness, and the Impossibility of Experience', *Journal of Ethics* 1 (1997), p. 345. If Fischer's account can be accepted (i.e. ER II can really be rejected as he believes), then it would *partly* support my point. However, to judge whether ER II is rejected by Fischer's example, an extensive discussion is needed. At least, it would be necessary to make clear what the term 'possible' in ER II means, or ought to mean.

14. 'Introduction: Death, Metaphysics, and Morality', in *The Metaphysics of Death*, ed. John Martin Fischer (Stanford: Stanford University Press, 1993), pp. 24-25.

15. In fact, Rosenbaum and Silverstein raise another problem for the deprivation theory. Rosenbaum, for instance, says:

> It is all right, I suppose, to call a person's death a loss for the person, but it is clearly not like paradigmatic cases of losses that are bad for persons. Consider the case in which one loses one's business to creditors. One has the business, the creditors get it, and then one does not have it. We may suppose that the loss is bad for the person. Such cases are common. We should note that in such cases the loss is something the person *is able to experience* after it occurs. Typical losses that are bad for persons seem to instantiate the following principle: A person P loses good g only if there is a time at which P has g and there is a later time at which P does not have g. If P ceases to exist when P dies, then being dead cannot be considered a loss of this typical sort in which losses are bad for persons, for in typical cases P exists after the loss and *is able to experience* it. If being dead is a loss, it is so insufficiently similar to paradigm cases of loss which are bad for persons that we need special reasons or arguments why treating death as a loss [which is bad for the person who dies]. (My emphasis.)

Stephen E. Rosenbaum, 'How to Be Dead and Not Care: A Defense of Epicurus', in *The Metaphysics of Death*, ed. John Martin Fischer (Stanford: Stanford University Press, 1993), p. 127. See also Harry S. Silverstein, 'The Evil of Death', in *The Metaphysics of Death*, ed. John Martin Fischer (Stanford: Stanford University Press, 1993), p. 100.

To this, we might reply, following McMahan and Sumner, as follows:

> Loss is bad for one. In most instances, it is true that the loss is something the person *is able to experience* after it occurs. But death is obviously a special case. That is, death is a special sort of loss (misfortune). It is special only because the subject and the object of the loss are identical. However, this fact should not rule out treating it as a loss (misfortune). To insist that it cannot be an evil because it does not meet a condition that most if not all other evils of loss satisfy is tantamount to ruling it out as an evil simply because it has special features.

See Jeff McMahan, 'Death and the Value of Life', in *The Metaphysics of Death*, ed. John Martin Fischer (Stanford: Stanford University Press, 1993), p. 241; and L. W. Sumner, 'A Matter of Life and Death', *Nous* 10 (1976), p. 160.

In fact, the real issue here is not 'whether or not we can call a person's death a loss for him'. That is, the real issue here is not about the appropriate use of the term 'loss'. I think that this issue is merely an appearance. In contrast, the underlying issue here is about the Existence Requirement. In other words, the debate here is the re-emergence of the above debate over the Existence Requirement in a slightly altered form. In his attack, Rosenbaum has, in fact, presupposed the Existence Requirement. Without rejecting Rosenbaum's presupposition, the reply here is actually begging the question. Thus, this reply does not really successfully refute Rosenbaum's attack. I think, the only appropriate way to successfully refute this attack is to reject the Existence Requirement. And this has already been done in Chapter One, Section Two.

16. See 'Death', in Thomas Nagel, *Mortal Questions* (London: Cambridge University Press, 1979), p. 9.

17. Ibid., pp. 8-10. In fact, Nagel also questions the imaginable view in the same paper. He says:

> We are left, therefore, with the question whether the nonrealization of this possibility [of our going on existing indefinitely] is in every case a misfortune [for us]...The question is whether we can regard as a misfortune any limitation, like mortality, that is normal to the species...the question remains whether death, no matter when it occurs, can be said to deprive its victim of what is in the relevant sense a possible continuation of life. (p. 9)

Basically, Nagel takes the imaginable view in this paper. After all, the imaginable view is consistent with the claim that death is *always* an evil.

18. Jeff McMahan, 'Death and the Value of Life', in *The Metaphysics of Death*, ed. John Martin Fischer (Stanford: Stanford University Press, 1993), p. 243.

19. See Ibid.

20. See Ibid.

21. Ibid., p. 244. This line of reasoning is also supported by Fischer. See John Martin Fischer, 'Death, Badness, and the Impossibility of Experience', *Journal of Ethics* 1 (1997), p. 347.

22. The reason for this is simply that life is *generally* good.

23. Jeff McMahan, 'Death and the Value of Life', in *The Metaphysics of Death,* ed. John Martin Fischer (Stanford: Stanford University Press, 1993), p. 245.

24. See Ibid.

25. See Ibid.

26. See Ibid.

27. See Ibid., pp. 245-246.

28. See Ibid., p. 245.

29. Ibid., p. 251.

30. Ibid.

31. Ibid., p. 252.

32. See Harry S. Silverstein, 'The Evil of Death', in *The Metaphysics of Death,* ed. John Martin Fischer (Stanford: Stanford University Press, 1993), p. 245.

33. See Jeff McMahan, 'Death and the Value of Life', in *The Metaphysics of Death,* ed. John Martin Fischer (Stanford: Stanford University Press, 1993), p. 253.

34. See Ibid., p. 245.

35. David K. Lewis, in discussing different ways of understanding counterfactual suppositions, refers to a wide delineation of the relevant facts. See David K. Lewis, *Philosophical Papers* (Oxford: Oxford University Press, 1986), p. 77.

36. In this case, it does not rule out the possibility that the doctor still sometimes feels that death is a harm to John. Alternatively he might have a compound feeling about John, and think that his death is a bad for him on the wider view but nevertheless see that it was a welcome release for him in the particular medical circumstances.

37. Jeff McMahan, 'Death and the Value of Life', in *The Metaphysics of Death,* ed. John Martin Fischer (Stanford: Stanford University Press, 1993), p. 248.

38. Ibid., pp. 249-250.

39. See Ibid., pp. 248-249.

40. See Ibid., p. 248.

41. It should be emphasised that, when evaluating a person's death, we sometimes, in a sense, single out the cause of his death as the closest one— the stop of the heart beat (by one common definition of death, if this definition is accepted). Or to put it in another way, we sometimes, when evaluating a person's death, completely ignore the cause of his death (though of course the death must have been caused *somehow*). That is, we, in fact, understand his death as merely the fact of his death at T. If we understand a person's death in this way, then, given the deprivation theory, the following conclusion would certainly be reached: Death is *generally* good for the person who dies. The reason is this. Most people will suffer awful pain due to sickness or accidents before they die. How many people can be as lucky as Albert Einstein who died in his sleep? This conclusion greatly conflicts the aim of the deprivation theory. In certain circumstances, it is easy or even very natural for us to evaluate a person's death in this way. But note that this is *not* the only way of evaluating a person's death. This suggests that the deprivation theory cannot apply for merely evaluating a person's death so understood. Given this, the deprivation theory would be more plausible and acceptable for us.

42. For convenience of expression, throughout the discussion of these cases, I always use a natural but loose description in evaluating a person's death. For instance, while evaluating Mort's death, I always say, 'Had he not died when and how he did, he would have lived a long life.' In fact, here what I really mean is that had he not died when and how he did, it is *highly probable* that he would have lived a long life. Indeed, it is imaginable that there is a person whose life is so unlucky that death (no matter how we specify the cause of it) would bring him a welcome release. For example, someone facing burning by his enemy might welcome a fellow soldier's fatal bullet. Because of these two reasons, the conclusion of the deprivation theory should be put as: Death is *generally* a harm to the person who dies (from a relatively wider view of the cause of his death).

43. According to the deprivation theory as developed so far, a person's death in his prime can even be a *good* thing for him in certain circumstances.

44. Jeff McMahan, 'Death and the Value of Life', in *The Metaphysics of Death*, ed. John Martin Fischer (Stanford: Stanford University Press, 1993), p. 247. For easier discussion later, what Joe further lost in being hit by the bus is changed from 'two months' to 'six months'.

45. See Ibid., p. 247.

46. For easy discussion, here I use the term 'death' in a loose way which refers to both death event and premature death. Strictly speaking, 'death' refers only to being dead.

47. By 'the death event', I mean a process from *the cause of death* to *death* (being dead) considered from a third-person or objective point of view. This should be distinguished from the process of *dying* discussed in Introduction, in which *dying* is to be understood as the first-person experience of the causal process which brings about death.

48. Feinberg, for example, supports this point. He says:

> If the prior interests set back by death justify our characterization of death as a harm (even without a subject), then equally some of them warrant our speaking of certain later events as posthumous harms. On the other hand, if the absence of a subject (even given prior interests whose targets postdate death) prevents us from speaking of death as a harm, then it equally precludes talk of posthumous harms. Death and developments after death are alike in coming into existence during a period when there is no longer a subject. If the absence of a subject precludes our speaking of posthumous harms, then equally it precludes our speaking of death as a harm...since both death and posthumous events are postpersonal. *Either death and posthumous harms both alike can be harms or neither can.* (My emphasis.)

Joel Feinberg, 'Harm to Others', in *The Metaphysics of Death,* ed. John Martin Fischer (Stanford: Stanford University Press, 1993), p. 174. Barbara Levenbook is also very convincing on this point. See Barbara Levenbook, 'Harming Someone after His Death', *Ethics* 94 (1984), pp. 407-419.

CHAPTER FOUR

1. Without any interest in Y, it is impossible for someone X to be harmed in virtue of any state of affairs concerning Y. In his article, 'Harm and Self-Interest', in *Law, Morality and Society: Essays in Honour of H. L. A Hart,* ed. P. M. S. Hacker and J. Raz (Oxford: Clarendon Press, 1977), p. 302, Feinberg makes a similar claim: 'It is only in virtue of having interests that people can be harmed...' Accordingly, it is concluded that the notion of harm relies on the notion of *interest.* Similarly, John Kleinig admits the importance

of the notion of *interest* for understanding the notion of harm. See John Kleinig, 'Crime and the Concept of Harm', *American Philosophical Quarterly* 15 (1978), p. 28.

2. See John Kleinig, 'Crime and the Concept of Harm', *American Philosophical Quarterly* 15 (1978), pp. 27-30.

3. Ibid., p. 28.

4. See Ibid.; and Joel Feinberg, 'Harm and Self-Interest', in *Law, Morality and Society: Essays in Honour of H. L. A Hart*, eds. P. M. S. Hacker and J. Raz (Oxford: Clarendon Press, 1977), pp. 285-286.

5. In Chapter Two, Section Two, I offer more illustration of the inconsistency between the concept of objective interest and the concept of desire.

6. It is not appropriate to explicate 'harm' as either the interference or the invasion of objective interests. For one thing, it is possible to interfere with or invade the objective interests of another without causing harm. Harm normally involves more than mere interference; it implies impairment. To impair something is to make it worse or cause it to deteriorate. See John Kleinig, 'Crime and the Concept of Harm', *American Philosophical Quarterly* 15 (1978), p. 32. For the remainder of this book I will use 'interest' to mean *objective* interest.

7. Joel Feinberg, 'Harm to Others', in *The Metaphysics of Death,* ed. John Martin Fischer (Stanford: Stanford University Press, 1993), p. 178.

8. In his book *Social Philosophy* (Englewood Cliffs: Prentice-Hall, Inc., 1973), p. 26, Feinberg says, '...harm is conceived as the violation of one of a person's interests...' Also in his article 'Harm and Self-Interest', in *Law, Morality and Society: Essays in Honour of H. L. A Hart*, eds. P. M. S. Hacker and J. Raz (Oxford: Clarendon Press, 1977), pp. 285-299, he writes, 'A person is [legally] harmed when someone invades (blocks or thwarts) one of his interests...'harm' [is] a violation of an interest ...'

9. See Joel Feinberg, 'Harm and Self-Interest', in *Law, Morality and Society: Essays in Honour of H. L. A Hart*, eds. P. M. S. Hacker and J. Raz (Oxford: Clarendon Press, 1977), pp. 287-290.

10. See Joel Feinberg, 'Harm to Others', in *The Metaphysics of Death,* ed. John Martin Fischer (Stanford: Stanford University Press, 1993), p.177. The distinction between fulfilment and satisfaction was made originally by W. D. Ross, *Foundations of Ethics* (Oxford: Clarendon, 1939), p. 300.

11. His reason for this claim is as follows:

Notoriously, fulfilment of desire can fail to give satisfaction...Indeed, the occurrence of subjective satisfaction is a highly contingent and unreliable phenomenon. Sometimes when our goals are achieved, we do not experience much joy, but only fatigue and sadness, or an affective blankness. Some persons, perhaps, are disposed by temperament normally to receive their achievements in this unthrilled fashion...Not only can one have fulfilment without satisfaction; one can also have satisfaction of a want in the absence of its actual fulfilment, provided only that one is led to believe, falsely, that one's want has been fulfilled...

Similarly, one's wants can be thwarted without causing frustration, or disappointment, and one can be quite discontented even when one's wants have in fact been fulfilled...A perfectly genuine and well-considered goal may be thwarted without causing mental pain when the desirer has a placid temperament or a stoic philosophy...One can have feelings of frustration and disappointment caused by false beliefs that one's wants have been thwarted, or by drugs and other manipulative techniques...

Most persons will agree, I think, that the important thing is to get what they want, even if that causes no joy. The pleasure that normally attends want-fulfilment is a welcome dividend, but the object of our efforts is to fulfil our wants in the external world, not to bring about states of our own minds.

Joel Feinberg, 'Harm to Others', in *The Metaphysics of Death,* ed. John Martin Fischer (Stanford: Stanford University Press, 1993), pp. 177-178.

12. See John Kleinig, 'Crime and the Concept of Harm', *American Philosophical Quarterly* 15 (1978), p. 33.

13. See Ibid., p. 31. For a deeper understanding of the notion of well-being, see J. David Velleman, 'Well-Being and Time', in *The Metaphysics of Death,* ed. John Martin Fischer (Stanford: Stanford University Press, 1993); Amartya Sen, 'Well-Being and Freedom', *Journal of Philosophy* 82 (1985), pp. 185-203; John Bigelow, John Campbell, and Robert Pargetter, 'Death and Well-Being', *Pacific Philosophical Quarterly* 71 (1990), pp. 119-140; and Michael A. Slote, *Goods and Virtues* (New York: Oxford University Press, 1983).

14. John Kleinig, 'Crime and the Concept of Harm', *American Philosophical Quarterly* 15 (1978), p. 31.

15. Ibid., p. 27.

16.   Ibid., p. 29.
17.   Ibid., p. 28. Feinberg also thinks that the rationality of the notion 'legal harm' can be doubted. See Joel Feinberg, 'Harm to Others', in *The Metaphysics of Death*, ed. John Martin Fischer (Stanford: Stanford University Press, 1993), p.180.
18.   See John Kleinig, 'Crime and the Concept of Harm', *American Philosophical Quarterly* 15 (1978), p. 29.
19.   Joel Feinberg, *Social Philosophy* (Englewood Cliffs: Prentice-Hall, Inc., 1973), p. 30.
20.   Ibid.
21.   To explain what 'in the way we normally lived (before)' means here, let us look back at John's case in Chapter Three, Section Two. In that case, if I state, 'The continuation of John's life in the way he normally lived (before)...', what I mean is: The continuation of John's life in the way he lived before this car accident. This should be emphatically distinguished from 'John's continuation of his life in excruciating pain'.
22.   Joel Feinberg, 'Harm to Others', in *The Metaphysics of Death*, ed. John Martin Fischer (Stanford: Stanford University Press, 1993), pp. 173-174.
23.   L. W. Sumner, 'A Matter of Life and Death', *Nous* 10 (1976), pp. 161-162. It is still in dispute whether life itself (or being alive) is a good or not. Some philosophers argue that it is. Nagel, for example, says:

> ...it is good simply to be alive, even if one is undergoing terrible experiences. The situation is roughly this: There are elements which, if added to one's experience, make life better; there are other elements which, if added to one's experience, make life worse. But what remains when these are set aside is not merely *neutral*: it is emphatically positive.

'Death', in Thomas Nagel, *Mortal Questions* (London: Cambridge University Press, 1979), p. 2. By contrast, other philosophers argue that life itself is *neutral*. Feinberg, for instance, says:

> There is something bare minimal about it [life itself] on the one hand, yet something supremely important on the other. Apart from the interests it [life itself] serves, it has no value in itself...

Joel Feinberg, 'Harm to Others', in *The Metaphysics of Death*, ed. John Martin Fischer (Stanford: Stanford University Press, 1993), p. 174. See also L. W. Sumner, 'A Matter of Life and Death', *Nous* 10 (1976), pp. 145-170. It is very important to resolve this dispute, particularly, when considering some issues about the choice between life and death from the utilitarian point of view. However, this is certainly not an easy task, and to do it is beyond the scope of this book. For the purpose of the discussion in this section only, it is enough to make sure merely that life is the precondition of a variety of goods.

24. John Bigelow, John Campbell, and Robert Pargetter also take this line of thought. They say, 'For a longer life will be a life of greater global well-being provided that the life in the extended period has a satisfactory character'. See John Bigelow, John Campbell, and Robert Pargetter, 'Death and Well-Being', *Pacific Philosophical Quarterly* 71 (1990), p. 136.

25. In fact, in the interest-impairment theory *of the harm of the death event*, I have combined the deprivation theory and the interest-impairment principle. It is true that the deprivation theory has correctly identified an important element for explaining why death *as an event* (from a relatively wider view of the cause of death) can be a *harm* to the person who dies. However, the deprivation theory omits the essential characteristics of *harm*. Strictly speaking, what makes death events (from a relatively wider view of the causes of death) *harms* to us is not the deprivation of certain goods—the goods we would have enjoyed if we had not died, as the deprivation theory maintains. It is rather because death events (from a relatively wider view of the causes of death) deprive us of certain goods and these goods are in our interests.

Similarly, it is not appropriate to say, 'Death as an event is a *harm* to us because it thwarts all our (future-oriented) dependent *unconditional* desires'. It would be more accurate to say, 'Death as an event is a *harm* to us because it thwarts all our (future-oriented) dependent *unconditional* desires and we all have an interest in not being thwarted in our desires'. After all, the thwarting of desires can sometimes be, on balance, good for us.

Here, I am not claiming that the deprivation theory is incorrect. What I claim is that the deprivation theory can be improved. In short, I suggest that to make the deprivation theory more appropriate, it should be supplemented with the interest-impairment principle.

26. In a sense, the continuation of our lives is *always* in our interests. For the continuation of our lives would *certainly* extend our lives which is in our interests. However, in excruciating circumstances, the interest in extending our lives might be regarded as relatively very trivial or unimportant and thus

ignored. After all, one of the essential reasons for a longer life is to enjoy it, not to suffer it.

27. Gisela Striker, 'Commentary on Mitsis', in *Proceedings of the Boston Area Colloquium in Ancient Philosophy*, vol. 4, eds. John J. Cleary and Daniel C. Shartin (New York: University Press of America, 1988), p. 325.

28. Ibid., pp. 325-326.

29. It seems to me that the notion 'completeness' is too vague to be used in this discussion. Particularly, it is not clear whether the notion 'completeness' has included the notion 'duration' or not. That is, it is uncertain whether or not 'to live a complete life' has already implied (or meant) 'to live at least the normal lifespan of a human being'. Indeed, it is doubtful whether it makes sense to say, 'A person has lived a *complete* life even if he only had a *short* life span'. However, for a strategic reason, I will reluctantly use this term for the discussion later. I want to show that even if I accept Striker's term, using her example, and following her line of reasoning, *duration* remains important in considering and evaluating the badness of premature death.

30. Again, for strategic reasons, I take her point concerning the notion of interest, which is roughly acceptable.

31. Gisela Striker, 'Commentary on Mitsis', in *Proceedings of the Boston Area Colloquium in Ancient Philosophy*, vol. 4, eds. John J. Cleary and Daniel C. Shartin (New York: University Press of America, 1988), p. 327.

32. Jeff McMahan, 'Death and the Value of Life', in *The Metaphysics of Death*, ed. John Martin Fischer (Stanford: Stanford University Press, 1993), pp. 254-256.

33. Joel Feinberg, *Social Philosophy* (Englewood Cliffs: Prentice-Hall, Inc., 1973), p. 30.

34. Ernest Partridge, 'Posthumous Interests and Posthumous Respect', *Ethics* 91 (1981), pp. 243-244.

35. See George Pitcher, 'The Misfortunes of the Dead', in *The Metaphysics of Death*, ed. John Martin Fischer (Stanford: Stanford University Press, 1993), p. 160.

36. See Ibid., p. 163.

37. See Joel Feinberg, 'Harm to Others', in *The Metaphysics of Death*, ed. John Martin Fischer (Stanford: Stanford University Press, 1993), pp. 180-181.

38. See Ibid., p. 176. It should be emphasised that what I mean by 'interest' here and thereafter is the *objective* interest as illustrated in this chapter, Section One. However, what Feinberg means by 'interest' is different from

what I mean which is inappropriately defined by (*objective*) desires. In his paper, 'Harm to Others', in *The Metaphysics of Death*, ed. John Martin Fischer (Stanford: Stanford University Press, 1993), p. 177, he says, 'As we have seen, interests are…derived from and linked to [*objective*] wants…' And also, in 'The Rights of Animals and Unborn Generations', in *Philosophical and Environmental Crisis*, ed. William T. Blackstone (Athens: University of Georgia Press, 1974), pp. 52-53, he says, 'Interests are compounded out of *desires* and *aims*…desires or wants are the materials interests are made of…'

39.   See Joel Feinberg, 'Harm to Others', in *The Metaphysics of Death*, ed. John Martin Fischer (Stanford: Stanford University Press, 1993), p. 179.

40.   See Ibid., p. 181.

41.   Rosenbaum and Partridge, for example, both take the same line of argument to reject the possibility of *posthumous harms*. See Stephen E. Rosenbaum, 'The Harm of Killing: An Epicurean Perspective', in *Contemporary Essays on Greek Ideas: The Kilgore Festschrift*, eds. Robert M. Baird, William F. Cooper, Elmer H. Duncan, and Stuart E. Rosenbaum (Waco: Baylor University Press: 1987), pp. 214-219; and Ernest Partridge, 'Posthumous Interests and Posthumous Respect', *Ethics* 91 (1981), pp. 246-253.

42.   Joel Feinberg, 'Harm to Others', in *The Metaphysics of Death*, ed. John Martin Fischer (Stanford: Stanford University Press, 1993), p. 183.

43.   Ibid., p. 176.

44.   George Pitcher, 'The Misfortunes of the Dead', in *The Metaphysics of Death*, ed. John Martin Fischer (Stanford: Stanford University Press, 1993), p. 161.

45.   Ibid. *Post*-mortem person strictly speaking is an oxymoron, because all *actual* persons are living and therefore *ante*-mortem persons. It would be less misleading to talk of *post*-mortem individuals, but I have followed the misleading usage of Pitcher and Feinberg in my exposition.

46.   Ibid.

47.   Joel Feinberg, 'Harm to Others', in *The Metaphysics of Death*, ed. John Martin Fischer (Stanford: Stanford University Press, 1993), pp. 183-184.

48.   See George Pitcher, 'The Misfortunes of the Dead', in *The Metaphysics of Death*, ed. John Martin Fischer (Stanford: Stanford University Press, 1993), p. 161.

49.   Raymond A. Belliotti, 'Do Dead Human Beings Have Rights?', *Personalist* 60 (1979), p. 203.

50.   Indeed, if death (being dead) is not a harm, then it would be implausible for us to claim that the *death event* (which brings about his death) is a harm. See Introduction, Assumption 4.

51.   Amelie Oksenberg Rorty, for example, also defends this position. She says, 'A harm must be a harm-to-someone; but if the dead are by definition extinct, they cannot be harmed by not existing.' Amelie Oksenberg Rorty, 'Fearing Death', *Philosophy* 58 (1983), p. 175. Similarly, Mary Mothersill says:

> Here there seems to be a contradiction. Assuming, as Nagel assumes, that Smith's death is a datable event, then, by definition, 'Smith is dead at time t' entails 'there is no time t+n subsequent to t such that at t+n there exists an x and x=Smith.'...Nagel says flatly that it is the individual who has died that is unfortunate. According to a familiar theorem of predicate logic, the sentence 'F of a' (where 'a' is a constant) implies 'There exists an x such that F of x and x=a.' Nagel's thesis, then, commits him to the following oddity: 'There is a time, t, such that at t Smith is unfortunate and there exists no such person as Smith.'

Mary Mothersill, 'Death', in *Moral Problems: A Collection of Philosophical Essays*, ed. James Rachels (New York: Harper & Row, Publishers, 1975), p. 373.

52.   As discussed above, clearly the well-being of a person's heirs can be in his interests. And these interests can survive his death, and thus be frustrated posthumously. Of course, the subject of these interests, and thus the corresponding harms would be the ante-mortem person. Given this, to fully secure a person's legal right, it might be the most reasonable way to devolve the properties of the deceased onto legal heirs (e.g. his son). Furthermore, a person can even decide to give all his property to a nursing home, but not to his own son. And this will be also protected by law. In a sense, my point can offer grounds for the common legal practice—devolving the properties of the deceased onto legal heirs. Thanks to the anonymous reviewer for emphasising this point.

53.   Julian Lamont, 'A Solution to the Puzzle of When Death Harms Its Victims', *Australasian Journal of Philosophy* 76 (1998), p. 198.

54.   See Ibid., pp. 198-212.

55. Fred Feldman, 'Some Puzzles about the Evil of Death', in *The Metaphysics of Death*, ed. John Martin Fischer (Stanford: Stanford University Press, 1993), p. 320.

56. Ibid., p. 321.

57. Julian Lamont, 'A Solution to the Puzzle of When Death Harms Its Victims', *Australasian Journal of Philosophy* 76 (1998), p. 199.

58. 'Death', in Thomas Nagel, *Mortal Questions* (London: Cambridge University Press, 1979), p. 7.

59. Julian Lamont, 'A Solution to the Puzzle of When Death Harms Its Victims', *Australasian Journal of Philosophy* 76 (1998), p. 208.

60. Ibid.

61. Ibid., pp. 208-209.

62. Ibid. p. 209.

63. Grey offers another version—the 'After Death' proposal—which also claims that the subject of harm by death is the *ante-mortem person*. We might, at the first glance, naturally suspect the plausibility of this version. We might ask, 'How can it be possible for a person to be harmed by death *after* his death? After all, P does not exist in any form at death and after. That is, there is no real subject of posthumous harms (and harm by death) left after his death.' However, it seems to me that Grey tries to answer a different question from mine. The timing question he answers is, 'When does the harm of death *accrue?*' This question is totally different from the question, 'When does someone's (P's) being harmed by death occur?' Perhaps, his question can be expressed as: When is the state of affairs that P was harmed by death made true from a third person perspective? Throughout this book, I want to focus on the solution to the missing subject problem raised by Epicurus. I therefore ignore Grey's question about the timing of the accrual of harm. See William Grey, 'Epicurus and the Harm of Death', *Australasian Journal of Philosophy* 77, (1999), pp. 358-364.

64. See Joel Feinberg, 'Harm to Others', in *The Metaphysics of Death*, ed. John Martin Fischer (Stanford: Stanford University Press, 1993), pp. 183-184; and George Pitcher, 'The Misfortunes of the Dead', in *The Metaphysics of Death*, ed. John Martin Fischer (Stanford: Stanford University Press, 1993), pp. 160-161.

65. Julian Lamont, 'A Solution to the Puzzle of When Death Harms Its Victims', *Australasian Journal of Philosophy* 76 (1998), p. 210.

66. Ibid.

67. Ibid., p. 198.

68.   See Ibid., p. 210; and John Martin Fischer, 'Hard-Type Soft Facts',
Philosophical Review 95 (1986), pp. 593-594.
69.   See Julian Lamont, 'A Solution to the Puzzle of When Death Harms Its
Victims', *Australasian Journal of Philosophy* 76 (1998), pp. 204-205.
70.   For more discussion of what appears to be some rather troublesome
implications of Feinberg's theory, see W. J. Waluchow, "Feinberg's Theory
of 'Preposthumous' Harm", *Dialogue* 25 (1986), pp.727-734.
71.   Marilyn Adams believes that a soft fact about a time is not fixed only by
what is true at that time but refers as well to facts which obtain at later times.
Joshua Hoffman and Gary Rosenkrantz take this point. However, they point
out that according to Adams' suggestion, no statement is a hard fact about any
time T. John Martin Fischer asserts that there are hard-type soft fact and soft-
type fact, and the two kinds of facts can both be fixed after later times. For
discussions of hard/soft fact distinction, see Marilyn Adams, "Is the Existence
of God a 'Hard' Fact?", *Philosophical Review* 76 (1967), pp. 492-503; John
Martin Fischer, 'Freedom and Foreknowledge', *Philosophical Review* 92
(1983), pp. 67-79; Joshua Hoffman and Gary Rosenkrantz, 'Hard and Soft
Facts', *Philosophical Review* 93 (1984), pp. 419-434; and John Martin
Fischer, 'Hard-Type Soft Facts', *Philosophical Review* 95 (1986), pp. 591-
601.
72.   Joel Feinberg, 'Harm to Others', in *The Metaphysics of Death*, ed. John
Martin Fischer (Stanford: Stanford University Press, 1993), p. 185.
73.   Ibid.
74.   Julian Lamont, 'A Solution to the Puzzle of When Death Harms Its
Victims', *Australasian Journal of Philosophy* 76 (1998), p. 203.
75.   Ibid., p. 204.
76.   Ibid., pp. 204-205.
77.   Some people might ask, 'But when exactly does someone's (P's) being
harmed by death occur?' To this question, Feinberg offers a general answer:
'At the moment he first acquired the interests that death defeats.' I think that
it might be very difficult (or even impossible) to decide when exactly he did
acquire these interests. But I doubt, as Pitcher points out, that there is, for our
purposes, any need to fix the precise time at which he first acquired these
interests and hence to fix the precise time at which his being harmed by death
occurred. Indeed, in support to the claim that the subject of 'the harm of
death' and 'posthumous harms' is the ante-mortem person, it is rather enough
to show, as I have done, that someone's (P's) being harmed by death or
posthumous events occurs *before* his death. See Joel Feinberg, 'Harm to

Others', in *The Metaphysics of Death,* ed. John Martin Fischer (Stanford: Stanford University Press, 1993), p. 186; and George Pitcher, 'The Misfortunes of the Dead', in *The Metaphysics of Death,* ed. John Martin Fischer (Stanford: Stanford University Press, 1993), p. 167.

78. To simplify discussion, in this section I discuss only the issue: *when* is someone (P) harmed (if it is a harm) by his own death? But note that all my points about this issue can also be applied to the timing of the harm of someone's (P's) premature death. That is, I suggest that P's being harmed by his premature death occurs *before* his death as well.

79. Chapter Four, Section Four is substantially based on my paper 'Commentary on Lamont's When Death Harms Its Victims', *Australasian Journal of Philosophy* 77 (1999), pp. 349-357. Thanks to Oxford University Press's permission.

CHAPTER FIVE

1. For a discussion of Lucretius' philosophical background, see Ronald E. Latham, 'Lucretius', in *Encyclopedia of Philosophy,* vol. 5, ed. Paul Edwards (New York: Macmillan, 1967), pp. 99-101.

2. Lucretius, *On the Nature of Things,* trans. H. A. J. Munro, in *The Stoic and Epicurean Philosophers,* ed. Whitney Jennings Oates (New York: Modern Library, 1957), p. 131. This elliptical argument has appealed to diverse philosophers throughout western philosophical history, such as Pseudo-Plato, Cicero, Seneca, Plutarch, Montaigne, Hume, and Schopenhauer. See Stephen E. Rosenbaum, 'The Symmetry Argument: Lucretius against the Fear of Death', *Philosophy and Phenomenological Research* 50 (1989), fn. 5.

3. Cf. Walter Glannon, 'Temporal Asymmetry, Life, and Death', *American Philosophical Quarterly* 31 (1994), p. 235.

4. Stephen E. Rosenbaum, 'The Symmetry Argument: Lucretius against the Fear of Death', *Philosophy and Phenomenological Research* 50 (1989), pp. 359-360. Some philosophers, such as David Furley, believe that the Lucretian symmetry argument is not at all directed to showing that it is not rational to fear death (as Rosenbaum's reconstruction of the Lucretian symmetry argument shows), but is rather used to reinforce the conclusion that nothing is good or bad for one who is dead. If they are correct in this point, then Feldman's reconstruction of the Lucretian symmetry argument would be more

appropriate than Rosenbaum's. However, I think that Rosenbaum has offered enough evidence to show that the Lucretian symmetry argument is directed against death anxiety during one's life. Even if Rosenbaum is wrong on this point, it is still appropriate for me to take his reconstruction of the Lucretian symmetry argument. For I will, in the following discussion focus mainly on premise (2) of Rosenbaum's reconstruction of the Lucretian symmetry argument. Premise (2) is essentially used to show that nothing is good or bad for one who is dead. That is, I can still grasp the point Furley makes about the Lucretian symmetry argument. See David Furley, 'Nothing to Us', in *The Norms of Nature: Studies in Hellenistic Ethics*, eds. Malcolm Schofield and Gisela Striker (Cambridge: Cambridge University Press, 1986), pp. 76-77; and Fred Feldman, 'F. M. Kamm and the Mirror of Time', *Pacific Philosophical Quarterly* 71 (1990), p. 23.

5. See 'The Makropulos Case: Reflections on the Tedium of Immortality', in Bernard Williams, *Problems of the Self* (Cambridge: Cambridge University Press, 1973), p. 82.

6. See Stephen E. Rosenbaum, 'The Symmetry Argument: Lucretius against the Fear of Death', *Philosophy and Phenomenological Research* 50 (1989), pp. 356-357.

7. In claiming that death is a harm, I am claiming that *in general* death is a harm. It may be that in particular circumstances death is a good thing, all things considered. Since this point has already been addressed, I am ignoring this possibility for the present discussion.

8. Temporal *attitude* symmetry (or asymmetry) is very different from temporal *value* symmetry (or asymmetry). Unfortunately, Glannon assimilates these two throughout his paper, 'Temporal Asymmetry, Life, and Death', *American Philosophical Quarterly* 31 (1994), pp. 235-236. In the introduction to this paper, Glannon points out that Nagel and other philosophers who adopt his view of death have raised an argument advocating temporal *value* asymmetry. Conversely, he claims, the Lucretian symmetry argument supports temporal *value* symmetry. Glannon believes that neither is sound. He therefore suggests a different temporal asymmetry argument. Apparently, the purpose of this paper is to suggest a temporal asymmetry argument to show a new temporal *value* asymmetry. However, while starting proceeding the text, he shifts the focus from temporal *value* asymmetry to temporal *attitude* asymmetry (by using the term 'asymmetrical rational concern'). But by the end of his paper, Glannon concludes all his discussion with a temporal asymmetry argument. The premise (2) of this argument—*the*

asymmetry thesis—is undoubtedly the heart of this argument, and is completely concerning temporal *value* asymmetry. Given this, I would interpret Glannon's discussion in this paper as follows. Glannon not only tries to suggest a temporal *attitude* asymmetry, but most importantly, also, as Fischer suggests, wants to explore a new temporal *value* asymmetry: Since we can (while we are alive) have unpleasant experiences as a result of things that happen in the prenatal environment, but we cannot have bad experiences after we are dead; prenatal nonexistence can be bad for an individual, but death is not. See John Martin Fischer, 'Death, Badness, and the Impossibility of Experience', *Journal of Ethics* 1 (1997), p. 351.

9. Walter Glannon, 'Temporal Asymmetry, Life, and Death', *American Philosophical Quarterly* 31 (1994), p. 238.

10. Ibid., p. 236. This quotation is originally from McMahan. See Jeff McMahan, 'Death and the Value of Life', in *The Metaphysics of Death*, ed. John Martin Fischer (Stanford: Stanford University Press, 1993), p. 234.

11. Walter Glannon, 'Temporal Asymmetry, Life, and Death', *American Philosophical Quarterly* 31 (1994), p. 238. For a more detailed understanding of the notion of the Existence Requirement, see Chapter One, Section Two.

12. See Ibid., p. 239.

13. See Ibid.

14. Ibid., p. 240.

15. Ibid., p. 242.

16. See Fred Feldman, 'Some Puzzles about the Evil of Death', in *The Metaphysics of Death*, ed. John Martin Fischer (Stanford: Stanford University Press, 1993), p. 308; and Harry S. Silverstein, 'The Evil of Death', in *The Metaphysics of Death*, ed. John Martin Fischer (Stanford: Stanford University Press, 1993), p. 98.

17. Anthony L. Brueckner and John Martin Fischer, 'Why Is Death Bad?' in *The Metaphysics of Death*, ed. John Martin Fischer (Stanford: Stanford University Press, 1993), p. 222.

18. See Ibid., pp. 222-223.

19. Ibid., pp. 223-224.

20. Derek Parfit, *Reasons and Persons*, relevant passage in *The Metaphysics of Death*, ed. John Martin Fischer (Stanford: Stanford University Press, 1993), pp. 193-194.

21. Anthony L. Brueckner and John Martin Fischer, 'Why Is Death Bad?', in *The Metaphysics of Death*, ed. John Martin Fischer (Stanford: Stanford University Press, 1993), p. 224. Rosenbaum also argues that Parfit's version

of the bias toward the future confuses 'preference' and such emotions as 'fear' and 'anxiety'. I do not want to discuss this issue here. See Stephen E. Rosenbaum, 'The Symmetry Argument: Lucretius against the Fear of Death', *Philosophy and Phenomenological Research* 50 (1989), pp. 364-365 and fn. 36.

22.   Stephen E. Rosenbaum, 'The Symmetry Argument: Lucretius against the Fear of Death', *Philosophy and Phenomenological Research* 50 (1989), p. 365.

23.   Ibid., p. 364.

24.   See Anthony L. Brueckner and John Martin Fischer, 'Why Is Death Bad?', in *The Metaphysics of Death*, ed. John Martin Fischer (Stanford: Stanford University Press, 1993), p. 227.

25.   Ibid.

26.   Ibid., p. 228.

27.   Ibid.

28.   Apparently, Parfit adopts the Prenatal-and-Posthumous harm approach. He writes:

> ...we are biased towards the future. Because we have this bias, the bare knowledge that we once *suffered* may not now disturb us. But our equanimity does *not* show that *our past suffering was not bad.* The same could be true of our *past non-existence...* (My emphasis.)

Derek Parfit, *Reasons and Persons*, relevant passage in *The Metaphysics of Death*, ed. John Martin Fischer (Stanford: Stanford University Press, 1993), pp. 205-206. This point is supported by Frances Myrna Kamm as well. She says:

> ...the Parfitian solution to the asymmetry problem presupposes that what happened in the past through prenatal nonexistence was just as *bad* for the person as what will happen because of his death in the future...*This explanation of our asymmetrical attitudes does not claim that death is worse than prenatal nonexistence because we care more about it.* (My emphasis.)

Frances Myrna Kamm, *Morality, Mortality: Death and Whom to Save from It*, vol. 1 (New York: Oxford University Press, 1993), p. 28. Kaufman also makes the same point as Kamm. He says:

In contemporary philosophical discussions about death there are two lines of responses to the symmetry argument. One...[is] initially proposed by Nagel...The second kind of response originated with Derek Parfit...on Parfit's view, our past non-existence might be *bad* after all, since it deprives us of good experiences, but we don't mind that. (My emphasis.)

Frederik Kaufman, 'Pre-Vital and Post-Mortem Non-Existence', *American Philosophical Quarterly* 36 (1999), pp. 5-7.

29. Anthony L. Brueckner and John Martin Fischer, 'Why Is Death Bad?', in *The Metaphysics of Death,* ed. John Martin Fischer (Stanford: Stanford University Press, 1993), p. 228.

30. See Ishtiyaque Haji, 'Pre-Vital and Post-Vital Times', *Pacific Philosophical Quarterly* 72 (1991), p. 173.

31. Ibid.

32. Although Nagel adopts the deprivation theory, he does not believe that prenatal nonexistence (or not being born earlier) is a deprivation of the goods of life. Thus, according to him, prenatal nonexistence is not a harm. I will discuss this below.

33. Anthony L. Brueckner and John Martin Fischer, 'The Asymmetry of Early Death and Late Birth', *Philosophical Studies* 71 (1993), p. 330.

34. Anthony L. Brueckner and John Martin Fischer, 'Why Is Death Bad?', in *The Metaphysics of Death,* ed. John Martin Fischer (Stanford: Stanford University Press, 1993), p. 228.

35. See Ishtiyaque Haji, 'Pre-Vital and Post-Vital Times', *Pacific Philosophical Quarterly* 72 (1991), p. 175.

36. See Anthony L. Brueckner and John Martin Fischer, 'Death's Badness', *Pacific Philosophical Quarterly* 74 (1993), p. 38.

37. Ibid., p. 40.

38. Ibid., p. 41.

39. Even if Brueckner and Fischer *do* adopt subjectivism, it seems that they still confront some difficulties. See Ishtiyaque Haji, 'Pre-Vital and Post-Vital Times', *Pacific Philosophical Quarterly* 72 (1991), pp. 176-177.

40. Ibid. p. 176.

41. See Ibid.

42. Anthony L. Brueckner and John Martin Fischer, 'Death's Badness', *Pacific Philosophical Quarterly* 74 (1993), p. 41.

43. As regards this point, Fischer says:

> If death is indeed a bad for the individual who dies, it is...[a bad] that cannot be 'read off' the temporally intrinsic states and properties of an individual at a time. Thus, it is not a 'current-time-slice' notion...Thus, whether a state or condition is a bad or misfortune may not depend solely on temporally *non-relational* or current-time-slice features of an individual. Rather, there is an interesting and important dependence on facts about *history* and *possibilities*. Death would thus be similar to other bads...in not having its normative properties issue solely from current-time-slice features. (My emphasis.)

'Introduction: Death, Metaphysics, and Morality', in *The Metaphysics of Death,* ed. John Martin Fischer (Stanford: Stanford University Press, 1993), p. 24. Nagel says also:

> ...it is arbitrary to restrict the...evils [e.g. death] that can befall a man to *nonrelational* properties...There are...evils [e.g. death] which are irreducibly *relational*; they are features of the *relations* between a person...and circumstances which may not coincide with him either in space or in time. (My emphasis.)

'Death', in Thomas Nagel, *Mortal Questions* (London: Cambridge University Press, 1979), p. 6.

44. See Frances Myrna Kamm, 'Why Is Death Bad and Worse than Pre-Natal Non-Existence?', *Pacific Philosophical Quarterly* 69 (1988), p. 162.

45. Ibid., p. 161.

46. Ibid., p. 162.

47. Ibid., pp. 162-163.

48. Although I concede that the Injury factor is a factor for the badness of death, I really doubt whether the mere *shapes* of events at the edges of life (i.e. the Insult factor and the Terror factor) can be any factors for the badness of death. For simplicity, I assume that both of these two factors are acceptable.

49. Frances Myrna Kamm, *Morality, Mortality: Death and Whom to Save from It,* vol. 1 (New York: Oxford University Press, 1993), p. 54.

50. 'Death', in Thomas Nagel, *Mortal Questions* (London: Cambridge University Press, 1979), pp. 7-8. Rosenbaum suggests that the issue is not whether one could have been *born* earlier, but rather whether one could have

been *conceived* earlier. If he is correct, Nagel's claim is best construed as the claim that it is not *logically* possible for a person to be, or to have been, *conceived* earlier. I take Rosenbaum's point in my discussion. See Stephen E. Rosenbaum, 'The Symmetry Argument: Lucretius against the Fear of Death', *Philosophy and Phenomenological Research* 50 (1989), p. 362.

51. Stephen E. Rosenbaum, 'The Symmetry Argument: Lucretius against the Fear of Death', *Philosophy and Phenomenological Research* 50 (1989), p. 361.

52. In his well-known book *Naming and Necessity,* Saul A. Kripke argues that personal identity requires an essentiality of origins, such as a particular genetic structure or some aspect of bodily continuity. He says, 'How could a person originating from different parents, from a totally different sperm and egg, *be this very woman?*...It seems to me that anything coming from a different origin would not be this object.' (p. 113). For more discussion of this topic, see Saul A. Kripke, *Naming and Necessity* (Oxford: Blackwell, 1980), pp. 111-116. Note that if Nagel's answer to Rosenbaum's challenge goes like this, 'There is an asymmetry between time of birth and time of death because time of birth is *essential* to us whereas time of death is not', then he begs the question.

53. See Stephen E. Rosenbaum, 'The Symmetry Argument: Lucretius against the Fear of Death', *Philosophy and Phenomenological Research* 50 (1989), pp. 362-363. Fischer also makes the same point. He says:

> Even if it is a necessary condition of personal identity that one issue from the particular sperm and egg cells from which one actually issues, this in itself would not imply that the particular time at which one is born is essential to personal identity. (Why couldn't those sperm and egg cells have existed earlier?)

'Introduction: Death, Metaphysics, and Morality', in *The Metaphysics of Death,* ed. John Martin Fischer (Stanford: Stanford University Press, 1993), p. 25. See also Anthony L. Brueckner and John Martin Fischer, 'Death's Badness', *Pacific Philosophical Quarterly* 74 (1993), fn. 2.

54. Anthony L. Brueckner and John Martin Fischer, 'Why Is Death Bad?', in *The Metaphysics of Death,* ed. John Martin Fischer (Stanford: Stanford University Press, 1993), p. 223.

55. In fact, Nagel himself also suspects that a person might be able to be born earlier. He writes:

We could imagine discovering that people developed from individual spores that had existed indefinitely far in advance of their birth. In this fantasy, birth never occurs naturally more than a hundred years before the permanent end of the spore's existence. But then we discover a way to trigger the premature hatching of these spores, and people are born who have thousands of years of active life before them. Given such a situation, it would be possible to imagine *oneself* having come into existence thousands of years previously.

'Death', in Thomas Nagel, *Mortal Questions* (London: Cambridge University Press, 1979), fn. 3.
56.   See Frederik Kaufman, 'Death and Deprivation; or, Why Lucretius' Symmetry Argument Fails', *Australasian Journal of Philosophy* 74 (1996), p. 307.
57.   See Ibid.
58.   Ibid., pp. 307-309.
59.   Ibid., p. 307.
60.   Christopher Belshaw also raises an argument for this point. See Christopher Belshaw, 'Asymmetry and Non-Existence', *Philosophical Studies* 70 (1993), pp. 109-112.
61.   Frederik Kaufman, 'Death and Deprivation; or, Why Lucretius' Symmetry Argument Fails', *Australasian Journal of Philosophy* 74 (1996), p. 309.
62.   Ibid.
63.   Ibid., p. 310.
64.   See Ibid., p. 311.
65.   See Ibid., p. 309.
66.   See 'Death', in Thomas Nagel, *Mortal Questions* (London: Cambridge University Press, 1979), fn. 3.
67.   Frederik Kaufman, 'Death and Deprivation; or Why Lucretius' Symmetry Argument Fails', *Australasian Journal of Philosophy* 74 (1996), pp. 309-310.
68.   Ibid., p. 310
69.   See Fred Feldman, 'Some Puzzles about the Evil of Death', in *The Metaphysics of Death,* ed. John Martin Fischer (Stanford: Stanford University Press, 1993), p. 322. Note that I am not here expressing the idea that being

born earlier is a bad for us. What I want to show here is that we do not really expect that being born earlier brings us more goods.

70. Michael de Montaigne, *Montaigne's Essays*, trans. Donald Frame (Stanford: Stanford University Press, 1958), p. 56. Montaigne is here paraphasing a remark made by Cicero. The thought goes back much further—at least to Socrates.

71. This idea has appealed to Pseudo-Plato, Cicero, Seneca, Plutarch, and Montaigne.

72. See Jeffrie G. Murphy, 'Rationality and the Fear of Death', in *The Metaphysics of Death*, ed. John Martin Fischer (Stanford: Stanford University Press, 1993), p. 44.

73. Baruch Spinoza, *Ethics and Treatise on the Collection of the Intellect*, trans. Andrew Boyle (London: Everyman, 1993), p.183

74. In his paper 'The Symmetry Argument: Lucretius against the Fear of Death', Rosenbaum illustrates this point clearly. He writes:

> When one thinks very deeply or reads very extensively about death anxiety [i.e. the fear of death], one is struck by its many faces. It is sometimes the fear of (painful) dying; sometimes the fear of the unknown; sometimes the fear of premature death; and sometimes the fear of nonbeing or nonexistence. It maybe, for some, an anxiety with no clearly identifiable object.

See Stephen E. Rosenbaum, 'The Symmetry Argument: Lucretius against the Fear of Death', *Philosophy and Phenomenological Research* 50 (1989), p. 354.

75. 'P's premature death' and 'P's death event (which brings about P's premature death)' are distinct. However, the latter would certainly lead to the former. Therefore, it seems that 'the fear of premature death' implies 'the fear of the death event (which brings about premature death)'.

76. O. H. Green, for example, argues that it is rational to fear death. On the other hand, Amelie Oksenberg Rorty, for instance, argues that it is irrational to fear death. Unfortunately, both of them confuse 'the fear of premature death' with 'the fear of necessary mortality'. See O. H. Green, 'Fear of Death', *Philosophy and Phenomenological Research* 43 (1982), pp. 99-105; and Amelie Oksenberg Rorty, 'Fearing Death', *Philosophy* 58 (1983), pp. 175-188.

77. Jeffrie G. Murphy, 'Rationality and the Fear of Death', in *The Metaphysics of Death*, ed. John Martin Fischer (Stanford: Stanford University Press, 1993), p. 49. Note that the expression 'P is rational in fearing' is ambiguous. On the one hand, we can mean that the *fear itself* is rational. On the other hand, we can mean that the *person* is rational in the *role* that he allows his fears to have in his life. What Murphy really means here by 'P is rational in fearing' is the latter one. See Ibid., pp. 47-48.

78. Ibid., 49.

79. Ibid. Mary Mothersill also explicates (2) as follows:

> One ground...for describing fear as 'irrational' is that it manifests itself in circumstances that the subject himself either knows or believes to be innocuous. For example, I am fearful of high places, lizards, mice, etc.

Mary Mothersill, 'Death', in *Moral Problems: A Collection of Philosophical Essays*, ed. James Rachels (New York: Harper & Row, Publishers, 1975), p. 380.

80. Jeffrie G. Murphy, 'Rationality and the Fear of Death', in *The Metaphysics of Death*, ed. John Martin Fischer (Stanford: Stanford University Press, 1993), p. 51. Rorty also illustrates (3) as follows:

> If fear of the horrors of dying from lung cancer...could be among the necessary causes of a person's taking steps to avoid that sort of death—his ceasing to smoking, changing his job or residence—then there would be good reasons for him to fear that sort of death. Indeed a person might judge that it would be wise for him to acquire that sort of fear, if doing so would lead him to take effective safety measures he is otherwise insufficiently motivated to take.

Amelie Oksenberg Rorty, 'Fearing Death', *Philosophy* 58 (1983), p. 176.

81. Jeffrie G. Murphy, 'Rationality and the Fear of Death', in *The Metaphysics of Death*, ed. John Martin Fischer (Stanford: Stanford University Press, 1993), p. 51.

82. 'The Makropulos Case: Reflections on the Tedium of Immortality', in Bernard Williams, *Problems of the Self* (Cambridge: Cambridge University Press, 1973), p. 82.

83. Of course, it is logically possible for one to live forever. However, it is practically impossible for him to live forever. After all, based on modern medical technology, immortality is (practically) impossible. In the discussion of ethical issues, I suggest taking the practical approach, instead of the logical approach.

84. See Jeffrie G. Murphy, 'Rationality and the Fear of Death', in *The Metaphysics of Death,* ed. John Martin Fischer (Stanford: Stanford University Press, 1993), p. 56.

85. Ibid., p. 52.

CONCLUSION

1. See Introduction, Assumption 4.

2. In claiming that death is a harm, I am claiming that *in general* death is a harm. It may be that in particular circumstances death is a good thing, all things considered. This point was considered earlier and I am ignoring this possibility for the present discussion.

3. See Hugh LaFollette, *Ethics in Practice: An Anthology* (Cambridge: Blackwell Publishers, 1996), p. 19.

4. See Ibid., pp. 66-68; and Thomas A. Mappes, 'Abortion', in *Social Ethics: Morality and Social Policy,* 3rd ed., eds. Thomas A. Mappes and Jane S. Zembaty (New York: McGraw-Hill Publishing Company, 1987), pp. 1-8.

BIBLIOGRAPHY

Ad Hoc Committee of the Harvard Medical School to Examine the Definition of Brain Death. 'A Definition of Irreversible Coma.' *Journal of the American Medical Association* 205 (1968): 337-340.

Adams, Marilyn. 'Is the Existence of God a 'Hard' Fact?' *Philosophical Review* 76 (1967): 492-503.

Agich, George J. 'The Concepts of Death and Embodiment.' *Ethics in Science and Medicine* 3 (1976): 95-105.

Agich, George J., and Royce P. Jones. 'Personal Identity and Brain Death: A Critical Response.' *Philosophy and Public Affairs* 15 (1986): 267-274.

Almeder, Robert. *Death and Personal Survival: The Evidence for Life after Death.* Lanham: Littlefield Adams, 1992.

Almog, Joseph, John Perry, and Howard Wettstein, eds. *Themes from Kaplan.* New York: Oxford University Press, 1989.

Annas, George J. 'Defining Death: There Ought to Be a Law.' *Hastings Center Report* 13 (1983): 20-21.

Annas, Julia. 'Epicurus on Pleasure and Happiness.' *Philosophical Topics* 15 (1987): 5-21.

Ayer, A. J. 'My Death.' In John Donnelly, ed. *Language, Metaphysics, and Death.* 2nd ed. New York: Fordham University Press, 1994.

Bataille, George. *Death and Sensuality.* New York: Walker, 1962.

Bealer, George. 'Review of Parsons' *Nonexistent Objects.*' *Journal of Symbolic Logic* 59 (1984): 652-655.

Becker, Ernest. *The Denial of Death.* New York: Free Press, 1973.

Becker, Lawrence C. 'Human Being: The Boundaries of the Concept.' *Philosophy and Public Affairs* 4 (1975): 335-359.

Belliotti, Raymond A. 'Do Dead Human Beings Have Rights?' *Personalist* 60 (1979): 201-210.

Belshaw, Christopher. 'Asymmetry and Non-Existence.' *Philosophical Studies* 70 (1993): 103-116.

Bennett, Jonathan. 'Counterfactuals and Temporal Direction.' *Philosophical Review* 93 (1984): 57-91.

Bernat, James L., Charles M. Culver, and Bernard Gert. 'Defining Death in Theory and Practice.' *Hastings Center Report* 12 (1982): 5-9.

Bigelow, John, John Campbell, and Robert Pargetter. 'Death and Well-Being.' *Pacific Philosophical Quarterly* 71 (1990): 119-140.

Boswell, James. 'An Account of My Last Interview with David Hume, Esq.' In *Private Papers of James Boswell* (Isham Collection).

Brandt, Richard. 'The Morality and Rationality of Suicide.' In Seymour Perlin, ed. *A Handbook for the Study of Suicide.* New York: Oxford University Press, 1975.

Brody, Howard. 'Brain Death and Personal Existence: A Reply to Green and Wikler.' *Journal of Medicine and Philosophy* 8 (1983): 187-196.

------------. *Ethical Decisions in Medicine,* 2nd ed. Boston: Little, Brown and Company, 1981.

Brueckner, Anthony L., and John Martin Fischer. 'The Asymmetry of Early Death and Late Birth.' *Philosophical Studies* 71 (1993): 327-331.

------------. 'Death's Badness.' *Pacific Philosophical Quarterly* 74 (1993): 37-45.

------------. 'Why Is Death Bad?' In John Martin Fischer, ed. *The Metaphysics of Death.* Stanford: Stanford University Press, 1993.

Bultmann, Rudolf. *Life and Death,* trans. P. H. Ballard, D. Turner, and L. A. Garrard. London: Black, 1965.

Callahan, Joan C. 'On Harming the Dead.' *Ethics* 97 (1987): 341-352.

Cameron, James M. 'On Death and Human Existence.' In John Donnelly, ed. *Language, Metaphysics, and Death,* 2nd ed. New York: Fordham University Press, 1994.

Capron, Alexander M., and Joanne Lynn. 'Defining Death: Which Way?' *Hastings Center Report* 12 (1983): 43-44.

Carter, W. R. 'Do Zygotes Become People?' *Mind* 91 (1982): 77-95.

------------. 'Once and Future Persons.' *American Philosophical Quarterly* 17 (1980): 61-66.

Cartwright, Ann, Lisbeth Hockey, and John L. Anderson. *Life Before Death.* Boston: Routledge and Kegan Paul, 1973.

Chisholm, Roderick M. 'Coming into Being and Passing away: Can the Metaphysician Help?' In John Donnelly, ed. *Language, Metaphysics, and Death,* 1st ed. New York: Fordham University Press, 1978.

------------. 'On the Observability of the Self.' In John Donnelly, ed. *Language, Metaphysics, and Death,* 2nd ed. New York: Fordham University Press, 1994.

------------. *Person and Object.* LaSalle: Open Court, 1976.

Cigman, Ruth. 'Death, Misfortune and Species Inequality.' *Philosophy and Public Affairs* 10 (1981): 47-64.

Clack, R. Jerold. 'Chisholm and Hume on Observing the Self.' *Philosophy and phenomenological Research* 33 (1973): 338-348.

Clarke, John J. 'Mysticism and the Paradox of Survival.' In John Donnelly, ed. *Language, Metaphysics, and Death,* 2nd ed. New York: Fordham University Press, 1994.

Cudd, Ann E. 'Sensationalized Philosophy: A Reply to Marquis's 'Why Abortion Is Immoral.' ' *Journal of Philosophy* 87 (1990): 262-264.

Crick, Francis. *Life Itself: Its Origin and Nature.* New York: Simon and Schuster, 1981.

Davis, Stephen T., ed. *Death and Afterlife.* New York: St. Martin's, 1989.

De Lacy, P. H. 'Epicurus.' In Paul Edwards, ed. *Encyclopedia of Philosophy,* vol. 3. New York: Macmillan, 1967.

Devine, Philip E. *The Ethics of Homicide.* Ithaca: Cornell University Press, 1978.

Diamond, Cora, and Jenny Teichman, eds. *Intention and intentionality.* Ithaca: Cornell University Press, 1979.

Donnellan, Keith. 'Speaking of Nothing.' *Philosophical Review* 82 (1974): 3-32.

Donnelly, John. 'Death and Ivan Ilych.' In John Donnelly, ed. *Language, Metaphysics, and Death,* 1st ed. New York: Fordham University Press, 1978.

------------. 'Eschatological Enquiry.' In John Donnelly, ed. *Language, Metaphysics, and Death,* 2nd ed. New York: Fordham University Press, 1994.

------------, ed. *Language, Metaphysics, and Death,* 1st ed. New York: Fordham University Press, 1978.

------------, ed. *Language, Metaphysics, and Death,* 2nd ed. New York: Fordham University Press, 1994.

------------. 'Suicide and Rationality.' In John Donnelly, ed. *Language, Metaphysics, and Death,* 1st ed. New York: Fordham University Press, 1978.

Ducasse, C. J. *A Critical Examination of the Belief in Life after Death.* Springfield: Illinois University Press, 1961.

------------. *Nature, Mind, and Death.* LaSalle: Open Court, 1951.

Eddin, Aron. 'Temporal Neutrality and Past Pains.' *Southern Journal of Philosophy* 20 (1982): 423-431.

Edwards, Paul. 'Existentialism and Death: A Survey of Some Confusions and Absurdities.' In John Donnelly, ed. *Language, Metaphysics, and Death,* 1st ed. New York: Fordham University Press, 1978.

------------, ed. *Immortality.* New York: Macmillan, 1992.

------------. 'My Death.' In Paul Edwards, ed. *Encyclopedia of Philosophy,* vol. 5. New York: Macmillan, 1967.

Enright, D. J., ed. *The Oxford Book of Death.* New York: Oxford University Press, 1987.

Epicurus. 'Letter to Menoeceus,' trans. C. Bailey. In Whitney Jennings Oates, ed. *The Stoic and Epicurean Philosophers.* New York: Modern Library, 1957.

Evra Van, James. 'On Death as a Limit.' *Analysis* 31 (1971): 170-176.

Ewin, R. E. 'What Is Wrong with Killing People?' *Philosophical Quarterly* 22 (1972): 126-139.

Falk, W. D. 'Morality, Self, and Others.' In Joel Feinberg, ed. *Reason and Responsibility: Readings in Some Basic Problems of Philosophy*. Belmont: Wadsworth Pub. Co., 1996.

Feifel, Herman, ed. *The Meaning of Death*. New York: McGraw-Hill Book Company, 1959.

Feinberg, Joel. 'The Forms and Limits of Utilitarianism.' *Philosophical Review* 76 (1967): 368-381.

------------. 'Harm and Self-Interest.' In P. M. S. Hacker, and J. Raz, eds. *Law, Morality and Society: Essays in Honour of H. L. A. Hart*. Oxford: Clarendon Press, 1977.

------------. 'Harm to Others.' In John Martin Fischer, ed. *The Metaphysics of Death*. Stanford: Stanford University Press, 1993.

------------. *The Meaning of Death*. New York: McGraw-Hill Book Company, 1959.

------------. ed. *Reason and Responsibility: Readings in Some Basic Problems of Philosophy*. Belmont: Wadsworth Pub. Co., 1996.

------------. 'The Rights of Animals and Unborn Generations.' In William T. Blackstone, ed. *Philosophy and Environmental Crisis*. Athens: University of Georgia Press, 1974.

------------. *Social Philosophy*. Englewood Cliffs: Prentice-Hall, Inc., 1973.

------------. 'Voluntary Euthanasia and the Inalienable Right to Life.' *Philosophy and Public Affairs* 7 (1978): 93-123.

------------. 'Wrongful Life and the Counterfactual Element in Harming.' *Social Philosophy and Policy* 4 (1986): 145-178.

Feldman, Fred. *Confrontations with the Reaper: A Philosophical Study of the Nature and Value of Death*. New York: Oxford University Press, 1992.

------------. 'On Dying as a Process.' *Philosophy and Phenomenological Research* 50 (1989): 375-390.

------------. 'F. M. Kamm and the Mirror of Time.' *Pacific Philosophical Quarterly* 71 (1990): 23-27.

------------. 'Some Puzzles about the Evil of Death.' In John Martin Fischer, ed. *The Metaphysics of Death*. Stanford: Stanford University Press, 1993.

Fischer, John Martin. 'Death, Badness, and the Impossibility of Experience.' *Journal of Ethics* 1 (1997): 341-353.

------------. 'Freedom and Foreknowledge.' *Philosophical Review* 92 (1983): 69-79.

------------. 'Hard-Type Soft Facts.' *Philosophical Review* 95 (1986): 591-601.

------------. ed. *The Metaphysics of Death*. Stanford: Stanford University Press, 1993.

Flew, Antony, ed. *Body, Mind, and Death*. New York: Macmillan, 1964.

------------. 'Can a Man Witness His Own Funeral?' *Hilbert Journal* 54 (1956): 242-250.

Foot, Philippa. 'Euthanasia.' *Philosophy and Public Affairs* 6 (1978): 85-112.

Foster, John. *The Immaterial Self: A Defense of the Cartesian Dualist Conception of the Mind.* London: Routledge, 1991.

Fulton, Robert, ed. *Death and Identity.* Bowie: Charles Press, 1976.

Furley, David. 'Nothing to Us?' In Malcolm Schofield, and Gisela Striker, eds. *The Norms of Nature: Studies in Hellenistic Ethics.* Cambridge: Cambridge University Press, 1986.

Geach, Peter. 'Immortality.' In John Donnelly, ed. *Language, Metaphysics, and Death.* 1st ed. New York: Fordham University Press, 1978.

Gervais, Karen Grandstrand. *Redefining Death.* New Haven: Yale University Press, 1986.

Glannon, Walter. 'Temporal Asymmetry, Life, and Death.' *American Philosophical Quarterly* 31 (1994): 235-244.

Glover, Jonathan. *Causing Death and Saving Lives.* New York: Penguin, 1977.

Green, Michael B., and Daniel Wikler. 'Brain Death and Personal Identity.' *Philosophy and Public Affairs* 9 (1980): 105-133.

Green, O. H. 'Fear of Death.' *Philosophy and Phenomenological Research* 43 (1982): 99-105.

Grey, William. 'Beginning and Ceasing to Exist.' *Philosophical Studies* 36 (1977): 393-402.

------------. 'Epicurus and the Harm of Death.' *Australasian Journal of Philosophy* 77 (1999): 358-364.

------------. 'Possible Persons and the Problems of Posterity.' *Environmental Values* 5 (1996): 161-179.

Griffin, James Patrick. *Well-Being: Its Meaning, Measurement, and Moral Importance.* Oxford: Clarendon Press, 1986.

Grover, Dorothy. 'Death and Life.' *Canadian Journal of Philosophy* 17 (1987): 711-732.

------------. 'Posthumous Harm.' *Philosophical Quarterly* 39 (1989): 334-353.

Hacker, P. M. S., and J. Raz, eds. *Law, Morality and Society: Essays in Honour of H. L. A. Hart.* Oxford: Clarendon Press, 1977.

Haji, Ishtiyaque. 'Pre-Vital and Post-Vital Times.' *Pacific Philosophical Quarterly* 72 (1991): 171-180.

Halley, M. Martin, and William F. Harvey. 'Medical and Legal Definitions of Death.' *Journal of the American Medical Association* 204 (1968): 423-425.

Hausman, David B., and A. Serge Kappler. 'Death as Irreversible Coma: An Appraisal.' *Journal of Value Inquiry* 12 (1978): 49-52.

Henson, Richard G. 'Utilitarianism and the Wrongness of Killing' *Philosophical Review* 80 (1971): 320-337.

Hick, John. 'Biology and the Soul.' In John Donnelly, ed. *Language, Metaphysics, and Death.* 2nd ed. New York: Fordham University Press, 1994.

------------. *Death and Eternal Life.* London: Collins, 1976.

------------. 'Towards a Theology of Death.' In John Hick. *God and the Universe of Faiths.* London: Macmillan, 1973.

High, Dallas M. 'Death: Its Conceptual Elusiveness.' *Soundings* 55 (1972): 438-458.

Hoffman, Joshua, and Gary Rosenkrantz. 'Hard and Soft Facts.' *philosophical Review* 93 (1984): 419-434.

Hoffman, Piotr. *The Human Self and the Life and Death Struggle.* Gainesville: University Presses of Florida, 1983.

Holland, R. F. 'Suicide.' In G. N. A. Vesey, ed. *Talk of God.* New York: St. Martin's, 1969.

Hull, Richard T. 'Some Reflections Occasioned by Clack and Chisholm.' *Philosophy and phenomenological Research* 35 (1974): 257-260.

Institute of Society, Ethics and the Life Sciences—Task Force on Death and Dying. 'Refinements in Criteria for the Determination of Death.' *Journal of the American Medical Association* 221 (1972): 48-53.

Ishiguro, Hide. 'Possibility.' *Proceedings of the Aristotelian Society* (supplementary) 54 (1980): 73-87.

Jantzen, Grace M. 'Do We Need Immortality?' In John Donnelly, ed. *Language, Metaphysics, and Death,* 2nd ed. New York: Fordham University Press, 1994.

Jonas, Hans. *Philosophical Essays: From Ancient Creed to Technological Man.* Englewood Cliffs: Prentice-Hall, Inc., 1974.

Jung, Carl C. 'The Soul and Death.' In Herman Feifel, ed. *The Meaning of Death.* New York: McGraw-Hill Book Company, 1959.

Kamm, Frances Myrna. *Morality, Mortality: Death and Whom to Save from It.* vol. 1. New York: Oxford University Press, 1993.

------------. 'Why Is Death Bad and Worse than Pre-Natal Non-Existence?' *Pacific Philosophical Quarterly* 69 (1988): 161-164.

Kaplan, David. 'Demonstratives.' In Joseph Almog, John Perry, and Howard Wettstein, eds. *Themes from Kaplan.* New York: Oxford University Press, 1989.

Kaufman, Frederik. 'Death and Deprivation; or, Why Lucretius' Symmetry Argument Fails.' *Australasian Journal of Philosophy* 74 (1996): 305-312.

------------. 'An Answer to Lucretius' Symmetry Argument against the Fear of Death.' *Journal of Value Inquiry* 29 (1995): 57-64.

------------. 'Pre-Vital and Post-Mortem Non-Existence.' *American Philosophical Quarterly* 36 (1999): 1-19.

Kaufmann Walter. 'Existentialism and Death.' In Herman Feifel, ed. *The Meaning of Death.* New York: McGraw-Hill Book Company, 1959.

Kleinig, John. 'Crime and the Concept of Harm.' *American Philosophical Quarterly* 15 (1978): 27-36.

Klemke, E. D. *The Meaning of Life*. New York: Oxford University Press, 1981.

Kluge, Eike-Henner W. *The Practice of Death*. New Haven: Yale University Press, 1975.

Koestenbaum, Peter. *The Vitality of Death: Essays in Existential Psychology and Philosophy*. Westport: Greenwood Pub. Co., 1971.

Korein, Julius, ed. *Brain Death: Interrelated Medical and Social Issues*. New York: New York Academy of Sciences, 1978.

Kripke, Saul A. *Naming and Necessity*. Oxford: Blackwell, 1980.

Kubler-Ross, Elisabeth, ed. *Death: The Final Stage of Growth*. Englewood Cliffs: Prentice-Hall, 1975.

------------. *On Death and Dying*. New York: Collier, 1993.

Ladd, John, ed. *Ethical Issues Relating to Life and Death*. New York: Oxford University Press, 1979.

Laertius, Diogenes. *Lives of Eminent Philosophers*. London: Heinemann, 1925.

LaFollette, Hugh, ed. *Ethics in Practice*. Cambridge: Blackwell Publishers, 1996.

Lamb, David. *Death, Brain Death and Ethics*. Albany: Croom Helm, 1985.

------------. 'Diagnosing Death.' *Philosophy and Public Affairs* 7 (1977): 144-153.

------------. 'Reply to Professor Wikler.' *Journal of Medical Ethics* 2 (1984): 102.

Lamont, Julian. 'A Solution to the Puzzle of When Death Harms Its Victims.' *Australasian Journal of Philosophy* 76 (1998): 198-212.

Latham, Ronald E. 'Lucretius.' In Paul Edwards, ed. *Encyclopedia of Philosophy*, vol. 5. New York: Macmillan, 1967.

Levenbook, Barbara Baum. 'Harming the Dead, Once again.' *Ethics* 96 (1985): 162-164.

------------. 'Harming Someone after His Death.' *Ethics* 94 (1984): 407-419.

Lewis, David K. *Counterfactuals*. Oxford: Blackwell, 1973.

------------. *Philosophical Papers*. Oxford: Oxford University Press, 1986.

Lewis, Hywel D. *The Self and Immortality*. New York: Seabury, 1973.

Li, Jack. 'Commentary on Lamont's When Death Harms Its Victims.' *Australasian Journal of Philosophy* 77 (1999): 349-357.

Lidz, Theodore. *The Person: His Development throughout the Life Cycle*. New York: Basic Books, 1968..

Lockwood, Michael. 'Singer on Killing and the Preference for Life.' *Inquiry* 22 (1979): 157-170.

Lucretius. *On the Nature of Things*, trans. H. A. J. Munro. In Whitney Jennings Oates, ed. *The Stoic and Epicurean Philosophers*. New York: Modern Library, 1957.

Luper-Foy, Steven. 'Annihilation.' In John Martin Fischer, ed. *The Metaphysics of Death.* Stanford: Stanford University Press, 1993.

Malpas, Jeff E. and Robert C. Solomon, eds. *Death and Philosophy.* New York: Routledge, 1998.

Mappes, Thomas A., and Jane S. Zembaty, eds. *Social Ethics: Morality and Social Policy.* 3rd ed. New York: McGraw-Hill Publishing Company, 1987.

Marquis, Don. 'Harming the Dead.' *Ethics* 96 (1985): 159-161.

------------. 'Why Abortion Is Immoral.' *Journal of Philosophy* 86 (1989): 183-202.

Martin, Raymond. 'Survival of Bodily Death: A Question of Values.' In John Donnelly, ed. *Language, Metaphysics, and Death.* 2nd ed. New York: Fordham University Press, 1994.

McInerney, Peter K. 'Does a Fetus already Have a Future-Like-Ours?' *Journal of Philosophy* 87 (1990): 264-268.

McMahan, Jeff. 'Death and the Value of Life.' In John Martin Fischer, ed. *The Metaphysics of Death.* Stanford: Stanford University Press, 1993.

------------. 'Preferences, Death, and the Ethics of Killing.' In Christoph Fehige, and Ulla Wessels, eds. *Preferences.* Berlin: W. de Gruyter, 1998.

Miller, Fred D., jr. 'Epicurus on the Art of Dying.' *Southern Journal of Philosophy* 14

(1976): 169-177.

Miller, Harlan B., and W. H. Williams, eds. *The Limits of Utilitarianism.* Minneapolis:

University of Minnesota Press, 1982.

Mitsis, Philip. *Epicurus' Ethical Theory: The Pleasures of Invulnerability.* London: Cornell University Press, 1988.

------------. 'Epicurus on Death and the Duration of Life.' In John J. Cleary, and Daniel C. Shartin, eds. *Proceedings of the Boston Area Colloquium in Ancient Philosophy,* vol. 4. New York: University Press of America, 1988.

Momeyer, Richard M. *Confronting Death.* Bloomington: Indiana University Press, 1988.

Montaigne, Michael de. *Montaigne's Essays,* trans. Donald Frame. Stanford: Stanford University Press, 1958.

Moody, Raymond. *Life after Death.* New York: Bantam, 1975.

Mothersill, Mary. 'Death.' In James Rachels, ed. *Moral Problems: A Collection of Philosophical Essays.* New York: Harper & Row, Publishers, 1975.

Murphy, Jeffrie G. 'Rationality and the Fear of Death.' In John Martin Fischer, ed. *The Metaphysics of Death.* Stanford: Stanford University Press, 1993.

Nagel, Thomas. 'Death.' In Thomas Nagel. *Mortal Questions.* London: Cambridge University Press, 1979.

------------. *The View from Nowhere.* New York: Oxford University Press, 1986.

Narveson, Jan. 'Future People and Us.' In Richard I. Sikora, and Brian Barry, eds. *Obligations to Future Generations*. Philadelphia: Temple University Press, 1978.

Nielsen, Kai. 'The Faces of Immortality.' In John Donnelly, ed. *Language, Metaphysics, and Death*. 2nd ed. New York: Fordham University Press, 1994.

Norcross, Alastair. 'Killing, Abortion, and Contraception: A Reply to Marquis.' *Journal of Philosophy* 87 (1990): 268-277.

Nozick, Robert. 'On the Randian Argument.' In Jeffrey Paul, ed. *Reading Nozick: Essays on Anarchy, State, and Utopia*. Oxford: Blackwell, 1982.

------------. *Philosophical Explanations*. Cambridge: Harvard University Press, 1981.

Nussbaum, Martha C. 'Mortal Immortals: Lucretius on Death and the Voice of Nature.' *Philosophy and Phenomenological Research* 50 (1989): 303-351.

Olson, Robert G. 'Death.' In Paul Edwards, ed. *Encyclopedia of Philosophy*, vol. 2. New York: Macmillan, 1967.

Parfit, Derek. *Reasons and Persons*. Oxford: Oxford University Press, 1984, relevant passage in John Martin Fischer, ed. *The Metaphysics of Death*. Stanford: Stanford University Press, 1993.

Parsons, Terence. *Nonexistent Objects*. New Haven: Yale University Press, 1980.

Partridge, Ernest. 'Posthumous Interests and Posthumous Respect.' *Ethics* 91 (1981): 243-264.

Paskow, Alan. 'The Meaning of My Own Death.' *International Philosophical Quarterly* 14 (1974): 51-69.

Penelhum, Terence. *Survival and Disembodied Existence*. London: Routledge & K. Paul, 1970.

Perrett, Roy W. *Death and Immortality*. Boston: Martinus Nijhoff Publishers, 1987.

Phillips, D. Z. *Death and Immortality*. Dordrecht: Nijhoff, 1987.

Pitcher, George. 'The Misfortunes of the Dead.' In John Martin Fischer, ed. *The Metaphysics of Death*. Stanford: Stanford University Press, 1993.

Plato. *Phaedo*, trans. Hugh Tredennick. In Edith Hamilton and Huntington Cairns, eds. *The Collected Dialogues of Plato*. Princeton: Princeton University Press, 1961.

Price, H. H. 'Survival and the Idea of 'Another World.' ' In John Donnelly, ed. *Language, Metaphysics, and Death*, 2st ed. New York: Fordham University Press, 1994.

Puccetti, Roland. 'The Conquest of Death.' In John Donnelly, ed. *Language, Metaphysics, and Death*, 1st ed. New York: Fordham University Press, 1978.

Quinn, Warren. 'Abortion: Identity and Loss.' *Philosophy and Public Affairs* 13 (1984): 24-54.

Quinton, Anthony. 'The Soul.' *Journal of Philosophy* 59 (1962): 393-409.

Rachels, James. *The End of Life: Euthanasia and Morality*. Oxford: Oxford University Press, 1986.

Rist J. M. *Epicurus: An Introduction*. Cambridge: Cambridge University Press, 1972.

Rorty, Amelie Oksenberg. 'Fearing Death.' *Philosophy* 58 (1983): 175-188.

Rorty, Richard. 'The Contingency of Selfhood.' *London Review of Books* 8 (1986): 11.

Quinton, Anthony. 'The Soul.' *Journal of Philosophy* 59 (1962): 393-409.

Rosenberg, Jay F. *Thinking Clearly about Death*. Englewood Cliffs: Prentice-Hall. 1983.

Rosenbaum, Stephen E. 'Epicurus and Annihilation.' In John Martin Fischer, ed. *The Metaphysics of Death*. Stanford: Stanford University Press. 1993.

------------. 'Epicurus on Pleasure and the Complete Life.' *Monist* 73 (1990): 21-41.

------------. 'The Harm of Killing: An Epicurean Perspective.' In Robert M. Baird. William F. Cooper, Elmer H. Duncan, and Stuart E. Rosenbaum, eds. *Contemporary Essays on Greek Ideas: The Kilgore Festschrift*. Waco: Baylor University Press. 1987.

------------. 'How to Be Dead and Not Care: A Defense of Epicurus.' In John Martin Fischer, ed. *The Metaphysics of Death*. Stanford: Stanford University Press. 1993.

------------. 'The Symmetry Argument: Lucretius against the Fear of Death.' *Philosophy and Phenomenological Research* 50 (1989): 353-373.

Ross, W. D. *Foundations of Ethics*. Oxford: Clarendon Press. 1939.

Sanders, Steven, and David R. Cheney. *The Meaning of Life: Questions. Answers and Analysis*. Englewood Cliffs: Prentice-Hall Inc.. 1980.

Sen, Amartya. 'Utilitarianism and Welfarism.' *Journal of Philosophy* 76 (1970): 463-489.

------------. 'Well-Being and Freedom.' *Journal of Philosophy* 82 (1985): 185-203.

Shaffer, Jerome. 'Persons and Their Bodies.' *Philosophical Review* 75 (1966): 59-77.

Sikora, Richard I., and Brian Barry, eds. *Obligations to Future Generations*. Philadelphia: Temple University Press. 1978.

Silverstein, Harry S. 'The Evil of Death.' In John Martin Fischer, ed. *The Metaphysics of Death*. Stanford: Stanford University Press. 1993.

Slote, Michael A. 'Existentialism and the Fear of Dying.' *American Philosophical Quarterly* 12 (1975): 17-28.

Smart, Ninian. 'Philosophical Concepts of Death.' In Arnold Toynbee, A. Keith Mant, Ninian Smart, John Hinton, Simon Yudkin, Eric Rhode, Rosealind Heywood, and H. H. Price, eds. *Man's Concern with Death*. London: Hodder & Stoughton. 1968.

Spinoza, Baruch. *Ethics and Treatise on the Collection of the Intellect*. trans. Andrew Boyle. London: Everyman. 1993.

Striker, Gisela. 'Commentary on Mitsis.' In John J. Cleary, and Daniel C. Shartin, eds. *Proceedings of the Boston Area Colloquium in Ancient Philosophy*. vol. 4. New York: University Press of America. 1988.

Sumner, L. W. *Abortion and Moral Theory*. Princeton: Princeton University Press. 1981.

------------. 'A Matter of Life and Death.' *Nous* 10 (1976): 145-171.

Swinburne, Richard. *The Evolution of the Soul*. Oxford: Oxford University Press, 1986.

Taylor, Charles. *Sources of the Self: The Meaning of the Modern Identity*. Cambridge: Harvard University Press, 1989.

Van Evra, James. 'On Death as a Limit.' *Analysis* 31 (1971): 170-176.

Veatch, Robert M. 'Brain Death.' *Hastings Center Report* 2 (1972): 10-13.

------------. 'Death.' *Theoretical Medicine* 5 (1984): 197-207.

------------. *Death, Dying, and the Biological Revolution: Our Last Quest for Responsibility*. New Haven: Yale University Press, 1976.

------------. 'Maternal Brain Death: An Ethicist's Thoughts.' *Journal of the American Medical Association* 248 (1982): 1102-1103.

------------. 'The Whole-Brain-Oriented Concept of Death: An Outmoded Philosophical Formulation.' *Journal of Thanatology* 3 (1975): 13-30.

Velleman, J. David. 'Well-Being and Time.' In John Martin Fischer, ed. *The Metaphysics of Death*. Stanford: Stanford University Press, 1993.

Wahl, Charles W. 'The Fear of Death.' In Herman Feifel, ed. *The Meaning of Death*. New York: McGraw-Hill Book Company, 1959.

Walton, Douglas N. *Brain Death: Ethical Considerations*. West Lafayette: Purdue University Press, 1980.

------------. *On Defining Death: An Analytic Study of the Concept of Death in Philosophy and Medical Ethics*. Montreal: McGill-Queen's University Press, 1979.

Waluchow, W. J. 'Feinberg's Theory of 'Preposthumous' Harm.' *Dialogue* 25 (1986): 727-734.

Wikler, Daniel. 'Correspondence: Brain Death.' *Journal of Medical Ethics* 10 (1984): 101-102.

Williams, Bernard. 'Egoism and Altruism.' In Bernard Williams. *Problems of the Self*. Cambridge: Cambridge University Press, 1973.

------------. 'The Makropulos Case: Reflections on the Tedium of Immortality.' In Bernard Williams. *Problems of the Self*. Cambridge: Cambridge University Press, 1973.

Woods, John. 'Can Death Be Understood?' In William R. Shea, and John King-Farlow, eds. *Values and the Quality of Life*. New York: Science History Publications, 1976.

Wreen, Michael J. 'The Definition of Death.' *Public Affairs Quarterly* 1 (1987): 87-99.

Wyschogrod, Edith, ed. *The Phenomenon of Death*. New York: Harper & Row, 1973.

Yourgrau, Palle. 'The Dead.' In John Martin Fischer, ed. *The Metaphysics of Death*. Stanford: Stanford University Press, 1993.

------------. 'On Time and Actuality: The Dilemma of Privileged Position.' *British Journal for the Philosophy of Science* 37 (1986): 405-417.

INDEX

Abortion. 137
Actual fact. 93-95
Afterlife. 1. 5. *See also* Soul
Ante-mortem persons. 8. 84-88. 91-92. 112-113
Asymmetry: between states of prenatal nonexistence and posthumous nonexistence. 101-103. 114-115. 117-119. 123-124

Backward causation. 87-88
Bad: comparative view of. 3-4
Being dead: 4-5. 13; death event and. 4-5
Belliotti, Raymond A., 86
Benefit. 72-74, 80-81
Bias toward future. 105-109
Brueckner, Anthony L. and John Martin Fischer. 106-113. 116

Categorical desires. 34-36
Causal overdetermination. 55, 59-64
Conditional desires. 34-35
Counterfactual conditionals. 50-53
Customary method of specifying the antecedent: arguments against. 50-52. 55-57; defence of. 54-59

Death: distinguished from dying. 2. 4. 13; concept of. 1-5. 44; common-sense view of. 1, 11; approaches to. 2-3; assumptions about. 1, 3, 5. 44; moral issues pertaining to. 1; metaphysical issues pertaining to. 1; anticipation of. 8. 16-17
Death event: distinguished from death. 4; concept of. 4. 6-7, 62-64; premature death and. 6-7. 62-64; harm of. 6-7. 74-77
Dependent desires. 35-36
Deprivation theory. 6, 43-44. 48-50. 58-59. 62, 64-65. 104. 109; arguments against. 44-47. 50-52. 55-56. 104-105; defence of. 45-48. 105-106; problems for. 6-7. 59-64; missing subject problem and. 2;

McMahan's critique of. 50-52; interest-impairment theory and. 77-78
Desire-thwarting theory. 6. 32-37; problems for. 6; arguments against. 37-41
Desires: concept of. 34-41. 68-69. 74-75; conditional. 34-35; categorical. 34-36. dependent. 35-36; independent. 35-36
Dying: distinguished from death. 2; 12-13; harm of. 2, 4

Epicurean argument. 2. 5. 11-19. 31; standard interpretation of. 12; assumptions in. 19-26; arguments against. 6. 26-31. *See also* Desire-thwarting theory; Deprivation theory; and Interest-impairment theory
Epicurus. 1-2. 5. 8. 11. 13-17. 20-21. 24-25. 99. 135
Euthanasia. 137
Evaluation: partial. 27; overall. 27
Evil: comparative view of. 3-4
Existence requirement. 6. 19-20. 46-47. 101-102; McMahan's critique of. 30-31
Experience. 17-18. 21
Experiential blank: death as. 2. 44. 46-47

Fear of death. 8-10. 124-125. 127-129
Fears: rational. 99-100. 123-127; irrational. 99-100. 125-127
Feinberg, Joel. 37-39. 68-70. 72-73. 75. 83-85. 91-95
Feldman, Fred. 88-89
Fischer, John Martin. 2-3. 13. 34. 36

Glannon, Walter. 101-104; critique of. 103-104
Grey, William. 73

Haji, Ishtiyaque. 109-111
Hard fact. 92-93
Harm: comparative view of 3-4; concept of. 7. 39. 67. 69. 74-75; moral. 71; legal. 71; Feinberg's definition of. 69-70; Kleinig's definition of. 70; prenatal. 101-103. 109

Immortality, 127; EM-type, 127
Impossibility, 22-23
Independent desires, 35-36
Interest-impairment principle, 7, 66-69;
    arguments against, 71; defence of, 72-73
Interest-impairment theory, 7, 66-88; of the
    harm of the death event, 75-78; of the
    harm of premature death, 79-80; of
    posthumous harms, 82-87
Interests, 68-69, 72-73, 79-81, 83-87;
    surviving, 83-87; self-regarding
    dependent, 83; desires and, 68-69
Irrational fears, 99-100, 125-127

Kamm, Frances Myrna, 113-114
Kaufman, Frederik, 9, 116-119, 121-123;
    critique of, 119-124
Kleinig, John, 68, 70-72

Lamont, Julian, 15, 87-93, 95-96; critique
    of, 88-97
Legal harms, 71
Life, 3, 75-76
Loss: death as, 43-44. See also Deprivation
    theory
Lucretian symmetry argument, 8-9, 47, 99-
    101; standard interpretation of, 100;
    arguments against, 101-109, 113-115,
    117-119, 123-124
Lucretius, 8-9, 99-100, 104, 113, 135
Luper-Foy, Steven, 35

McMahan, Jeff, 5, 30, 48-50, 52-59, 80
McMahan's method of specifying the
    antecedent, 52-53, 55-57; arguments
    against, 53-58
Misfortune: comparative view of, 3-4
Missing subject problem, 2, 7-8, 83-84, 87;
    concerning posthumous harms, 83-84;
    concerning the harm of death, 87;
    deprivation theory and, 2
Montaigne, Michael de, 124
Moral harms, 71
Mortality, 127-128; fear of, 127-128
Murphy, Jeffrie G., 125-126, 128

Nagel, Thomas, 9, 27, 43, 45, 48-50, 89-90,
    108, 114-116; McMahan's critique of,

48-50; Rosenbaum's critique of, 115-
    116; Brueckner and Fischer's critique of,
    116
Nozick, Robert, 45, 120

Objectivism, 111

Parfit, Derek, 40, 105-108; critique of, 106-
    107
Partridge, Ernest, 81
Personal identity, 5, 114-116
Pitcher, George, 29, 84-85, 91, 94
Plato, 1
Possible goods account, see Deprivation
    theory
Posthumous harms, 7, 64, 82-87; subject of,
    83-86; harm of the death event and, 7,
    64
Posthumous nonexistence, 8, 47, 99-115.
    See also Death
Post-mortem persons, 85-86, 91
Potential fact, 93-95
Premature death, 6-7, 61-62, 128; harm of 7,
    61-62; fear of, 128-129
Prenatal events, 102
Prenatal nonexistence, 9, 47, 99-105, 107-
    108, 123
Prenatal harms, 101-103, 109
Problem of specifying the antecedent, 50-52

Rational fears, 99-100, 123-127
Rosenbaum, Stephen E., 4, 13-15, 17-18,
    21, 23-24, 41, 46, 100, 106-107, 115-
    116

Silverstein, Harry S., 11, 43
Soft fact, 92-93
Soul, 1, 5. See also Afterlife
Specifying the antecedent: problems of, 50-
    52; McMahan's method of, 52-53, 55-
    56; customary method of, 50-52, 54-59
Spinoza, Baruch, 124
Striker, Gisela, 78-79; critique of, 79
Subjectivism, 111
Summer, L. S., 44, 76

Third stage intervening between dying and
    death, 4, 13-16

Timing of the harm of death, 8, 88-97;
    'Eternal' version of, 88-89; 'At No
    Time' version of, 89-91; 'At Death'
    version of, 91-92; 'Before Death' version
    of, 92-97
Transitive cause, 52

Welfare, 70
Williams, Bernard, 33-35, 43, 100, 126-127

Philosophy and Medicine

1. H. Tristram Engelhardt, Jr. and S.F. Spicker (eds.): *Evaluation and Explanation in the Biomedical Sciences.* 1975   ISBN 90-277-0553-4
2. S.F. Spicker and H. Tristram Engelhardt, Jr. (eds.): *Philosophical Dimensions of the Neuro-Medical Sciences.* 1976   ISBN 90-277-0672-7
3. S.F. Spicker and H. Tristram Engelhardt, Jr. (eds.): *Philosophical Medical Ethics.* Its Nature and Significance. 1977   ISBN 90-277-0772-3
4. H. Tristram Engelhardt, Jr. and S.F. Spicker (eds.): *Mental Health.* Philosophical Perspectives. 1978   ISBN 90-277-0828-2
5. B.A. Brody and H. Tristram Engelhardt, Jr. (eds.): *Mental Illness.* Law and Public Policy. 1980   ISBN 90-277-1057-0
6. H. Tristram Engelhardt, Jr., S.F. Spicker and B. Towers (eds.): *Clinical Judgment.* A Critical Appraisal. 1979   ISBN 90-277-0952-1
7. S.F. Spicker (ed.): *Organism, Medicine, and Metaphysics.* Essays in Honor of Hans Jonas on His 75th Birthday. 1978   ISBN 90-277-0823-1
8. E.E. Shelp (ed.): *Justice and Health Care.* 1981
                    ISBN 90-277-1207-7; Pb 90-277-1251-4
9. S.F. Spicker, J.M. Healey, Jr. and H. Tristram Engelhardt, Jr. (eds.): *The Law-Medicine Relation.* A Philosophical Exploration. 1981   ISBN 90-277-1217-4
10. W.B. Bondeson, H. Tristram Engelhardt, Jr., S.F. Spicker and J.M. White, Jr. (eds.): *New Knowledge in the Biomedical Sciences.* Some Moral Implications of Its Acquisition, Possession, and Use. 1982   ISBN 90-277-1319-7
11. E.E. Shelp (ed.): *Beneficence and Health Care.* 1982   ISBN 90-277-1377-4
12. G.J. Agich (ed.): *Responsibility in Health Care.* 1982   ISBN 90-277-1417-7
13. W.B. Bondeson, H. Tristram Engelhardt, Jr., S.F. Spicker and D.H. Winship: *Abortion and the Status of the Fetus.* 2nd printing, 1984   ISBN 90-277-1493-2
14. E.E. Shelp (ed.): *The Clinical Encounter.* The Moral Fabric of the Patient-Physician Relationship. 1983   ISBN 90-277-1593-9
15. L. Kopelman and J.C. Moskop (eds.): *Ethics and Mental Retardation.* 1984
                    ISBN 90-277-1630-7
16. L. Nordenfelt and B.I.B. Lindahl (eds.): *Health, Disease, and Causal Explanations in Medicine.* 1984   ISBN 90-277-1660-9
17. E.E. Shelp (ed.): *Virtue and Medicine.* Explorations in the Character of Medicine. 1985   ISBN 90-277-1808-3
18. P. Carrick: *Medical Ethics in Antiquity.* Philosophical Perspectives on Abortion and Euthanasia. 1985   ISBN 90-277-1825-3; Pb 90-277-1915-2
19. J.C. Moskop and L. Kopelman (eds.): *Ethics and Critical Care Medicine.* 1985
                    ISBN 90-277-1820-2
20. E.E. Shelp (ed.): *Theology and Bioethics.* Exploring the Foundations and Frontiers. 1985   ISBN 90-277-1857-1

Philosophy and Medicine

21. G.J. Agich and C.E. Begley (eds.): *The Price of Health.* 1986
ISBN 90-277-2285-4
22. E.E. Shelp (ed.): *Sexuality and Medicine.* Vol. I: Conceptual Roots. 1987
ISBN 90-277-2290-0; Pb 90-277-2386-9
23. E.E. Shelp (ed.): *Sexuality and Medicine.* Vol. II: Ethical Viewpoints in Transition.
1987 ISBN 1-55608-013-1; Pb 1-55608-016-6
24. R.C. McMillan, H. Tristram Engelhardt, Jr., and S.F. Spicker (eds.): *Euthanasia and the Newborn.* Conflicts Regarding Saving Lives. 1987
ISBN 90-277-2299-4; Pb 1-55608-039-5
25. S.F. Spicker, S.R. Ingman and I.R. Lawson (eds.): *Ethical Dimensions of Geriatric Care.* Value Conflicts for the 21th Century. 1987 ISBN 1-55608-027-1
26. L. Nordenfelt: *On the Nature of Health.* An Action-Theoretic Approach. 2nd, rev. ed. 1995 SBN 0-7923-3369-1; Pb 0-7923-3470-1
27. S.F. Spicker, W.B. Bondeson and H. Tristram Engelhardt, Jr. (eds.): *The Contraceptive Ethos.* Reproductive Rights and Responsibilities. 1987
ISBN 1-55608-035-2
28. S.F. Spicker, I. Alon, A. de Vries and H. Tristram Engelhardt, Jr. (eds.): *The Use of Human Beings in Research.* With Special Reference to Clinical Trials. 1988
ISBN 1-55608-043-3
29. N.M.P. King, L.R. Churchill and A.W. Cross (eds.): *The Physician as Captain of the Ship.* A Critical Reappraisal. 1988 ISBN 1-55608-044-1
30. H.-M. Sass and R.U. Massey (eds.): *Health Care Systems.* Moral Conflicts in European and American Public Policy. 1988 ISBN 1-55608-045-X
31. R.M. Zaner (ed.): *Death: Beyond Whole-Brain Criteria.* 1988
ISBN 1-55608-053-0
32. B.A. Brody (ed.): *Moral Theory and Moral Judgments in Medical Ethics.* 1988
ISBN 1-55608-060-3
33. L.M. Kopelman and J.C. Moskop (eds.): *Children and Health Care.* Moral and Social Issues. 1989 ISBN 1-55608-078-6
34. E.D. Pellegrino, J.P. Langan and J. Collins Harvey (eds.): *Catholic Perspectives on Medical Morals.* Foundational Issues. 1989 ISBN 1-55608-083-2
35. B.A. Brody (ed.): *Suicide and Euthanasia.* Historical and Contemporary Themes.
1989 ISBN 0-7923-0106-4
36. H.A.M.J. ten Have, G.K. Kimsma and S.F. Spicker (eds.): *The Growth of Medical Knowledge.* 1990 ISBN 0-7923-0736-4
37. I. Löwy (ed.): *The Polish School of Philosophy of Medicine.* From Tytus Chałubiński (1820–1889) to Ludwik Fleck (1896–1961). 1990
ISBN 0-7923-0958-8
38. T.J. Bole III and W.B. Bondeson: *Rights to Health Care.* 1991
ISBN 0-7923-1137-X

Philosophy and Medicine

39. M.A.G. Cutter and E.E. Shelp (eds.): *Competency. A Study of Informal Competency Determinations in Primary Care.* 1991   ISBN 0-7923-1304-6
40. J.L. Peset and D. Gracia (eds.): *The Ethics of Diagnosis.* 1992
                                                                    ISBN 0-7923-1544-8
41. K.W. Wildes, S.J., F. Abel, S.J. and J.C. Harvey (eds.): *Birth, Suffering, and Death.* Catholic Perspectives at the Edges of Life. 1992 [CSiB-1]
                                              ISBN 0-7923-1547-2; Pb 0-7923-2545-1
42. S.K. Toombs: *The Meaning of Illness.* A Phenomenological Account of the Different Perspectives of Physician and Patient. 1992
                                              ISBN 0-7923-1570-7; Pb 0-7923-2443-9
43. D. Leder (ed.): *The Body in Medical Thought and Practice.* 1992
                                                                    ISBN 0-7923-1657-6
44. C. Delkeskamp-Hayes and M.A.G. Cutter (eds.): *Science, Technology, and the Art of Medicine.* European-American Dialogues. 1993   ISBN 0-7923-1869-2
45. R. Baker, D. Porter and R. Porter (eds.): *The Codification of Medical Morality.* Historical and Philosophical Studies of the Formalization of Western Medical Morality in the 18th and 19th Centuries, Volume One: Medical Ethics and Etiquette in the 18th Century. 1993   ISBN 0-7923-1921-4
46. K. Bayertz (ed.): *The Concept of Moral Consensus.* The Case of Technological Interventions in Human Reproduction. 1994   ISBN 0-7923-2615-6
47. L. Nordenfelt (ed.): *Concepts and Measurement of Quality of Life in Health Care.* 1994 [ESiP-1]   ISBN 0-7923-2824-8
48. R. Baker and M.A. Strosberg (eds.) with the assistance of J. Bynum: *Legislating Medical Ethics.* A Study of the New York State Do-Not-Resuscitate Law. 1995
                                                                    ISBN 0-7923-2995-3
49. R. Baker (ed.): *The Codification of Medical Morality.* Historical and Philosophical Studies of the Formalization of Western Morality in the 18th and 19th Centuries, Volume Two: Anglo-American Medical Ethics and Medical Jurisprudence in the 19th Century. 1995   ISBN 0-7923-3528-7; Pb 0-7923-3529-5
50. R.A. Carson and C.R. Burns (eds.): *Philosophy of Medicine and Bioethics.* A Twenty-Year Retrospective and Critical Appraisal. 1997 ISBN 0-7923-3545-7
51. K.W. Wildes, S.J. (ed.): *Critical Choices and Critical Care.* Catholic Perspectives on Allocating Resources in Intensive Care Medicine. 1995 [CSiB-2]
                                                                    ISBN 0-7923-3382-9
52. K. Bayertz (ed.): *Sanctity of Life and Human Dignity.* 1996
                                                                    ISBN 0-7923-3739-5
53. Kevin Wm. Wildes, S.J. (ed.): *Infertility: A Crossroad of Faith, Medicine, and Technology.* 1996   ISBN 0-7923-4061-2
54. Kazumasa Hoshino (ed.): *Japanese and Western Bioethics.* Studies in Moral Diversity. 1996   ISBN 0-7923-4112-0